AN
IMMENSE
NEW
POWER
TO
HEAL

THE PROMISE OF PERSONALIZED MEDICINE

AN
IMMENSE
NEW
POWER
TO
HEAL

THE PROMISE OF PERSONALIZED MEDICINE

LEE GUTKIND
& PAGAN KENNEDY

In Fact Books
Pittsburgh

Requests for permission to reproduce material
from this work should be sent to:

Rights and Permissions
In Fact Books
c/o Creative Nonfiction Books
Creative Nonfiction Foundation
5501 Walnut Street, Suite 202
Pittsburgh, PA 15232

Cover design by Tristen Knight
Interior design by Heidi Whitcomb

ISBN: 978-1-9371630-6-8

Printed in the United States of America

The parts of this book primarily relating to the patient advocacy movement, including the chapters about PatientsLikeMe, ePatient Dave deBronkart, and personal medical devices, were written by Pagan Kennedy.

The authors wish to thank the Virginia G. Piper Charitable Trust and Judy Jolley Mohraz, its Chief Executive Officer and President, for support and cooperation during the time this book has been in progress. The Virginia G. Piper Charitable Trust is a foundation devoted to the approximately 4 million residents of Maricopa County, Arizona, a region that includes Phoenix, Tempe, and Scottsdale. The Trust has many interests, including arts and culture, children, older adults, education and religious organizations, along with healthcare and cutting edge medical research, to which they have contributed generously in the Maricopa County community.

TABLE OF CONTENTS

"With this profound new knowledge, humankind is on the verge of gaining immense, new power to heal. Genome science will have a real impact on all our lives—and even more, on the lives of our children. It will revolutionize the diagnosis, prevention, and treatment of most, if not all, human diseases."

—President Bill Clinton,
announcing the sequencing of the human genome, June 26, 2000.

INTRODUCTION:
EL DORADO OR IRON PYRITE?

Smiling and sipping nervously from a paper Starbucks cup, Dr. Lawrence Brody begins his lecture by providing three intriguing examples of personalized medicine. One, he says, is achievable today; the others are, in some ways, "futuristic." He doesn't tell us which is which—it's kind of a guessing game, perhaps like personalized medicine itself.

Brody is chief and senior investigator in the Genome Technology Branch of the National Human Genome Research Institute at the National Institutes of Health (NIH), and the title of his talk reflects some uncertainty about the state of his field: "Genetics & Personalized Medicine: El Dorado or Iron Pyrite? Will Personalized Medicine Live Up to the Hype?" El Dorado, of course, is the mythical lost city of gold, and iron pyrite is fool's gold. At the beginning of his talk, Brody puts a sample of the latter into circulation around the room, and as audience members pass the nugget to one another, the golden specks glint and glitter deceptively.

The first scenario concerns a 60-year-old man who takes a test that screens his prostate. The test is not the routine (and controversial) PSA, but a more precise diagnostic tool that has been developed from biomarkers—cell molecules that provide clues to genetic traits or disease. The test indicates high risk, and the doctors recommend—and the man subsequently agrees to—a biopsy. The news is not good. The biopsy reveals a cancerous tumor on the man's prostate.

Before recommending intervention, the doctors examine the genetic make-up of the tumor to try to predict whether it is likely to metastasize—"and maybe kill him," Brody adds. Based upon the genetic information, the doctors recognize the danger inherent in the tumor, scour their arsenal and choose or devise a drug tailored to eradicate that particular kind of cancer. Thus, they will eliminate the danger, complications and expense of surgery and the inevitably awful side effects of massive chemotherapy. The drug cures the man—a happy ending.

Someday, all cancer may be eradicated with the help of this sort of genetic testing. In fact, as awesome as it is to contemplate curing cancer, that's only a beginning: genetic testing techniques are advancing so rapidly that doctors may soon be able to administer exams to find out which types of medicine would work best for many more diseases—from diabetes to heart disease, and perhaps even the common cold!

In the second scenario, a ten-year-old girl's genome is scanned, and she is determined to be at very high risk for developing lung cancer. The scan also reveals that she carries three of the strongest genetic predictors for having an addictive personality. In a way, you could say the girl is genetically programmed for disaster.

This genetic information is provided to the girl's junior high school counselor and shared with administrators and teachers. Consequently, throughout her teen years, the girl is specifically targeted with antismoking interventions, including literature and persuasive conversations. Most smokers start young; but if this girl makes it to twenty-five without smoking, the odds are she will be out of the danger zone, Brody says, significantly reducing her risk of developing lung cancer. So here's another potential success story. Though we don't know about other ramifications of the girl's potentially addictive personality, we can assume that similarly appropriate actions will have been instituted to improve her chances of a less troubled life.

This is one of the advantages and goals of personalized medicine, Brody explains. Genetic information can predict the future—and thus can lead to early diagnoses that may minimize invasive procedures and allow physicians to more accurately prescribe drugs and help patients modify their behavior. Brody and his colleagues around the world envision a future in which personalized medicine is practiced in this manner, improving patient care immeasurably.

And yet, the personalized medicine movement is not only about patient health; it is also about the potential health of the economy. The successful realization and adoption of personalized medicine techniques would result in a massive shift in the allocation of resources that would inevitably lead to a total transformation of our out-of-control healthcare system. This is the reason so many scientists and government officials find personalized medicine attractive and compelling: potentially, it will help save trillions of dollars. It might also help fortify the scientific community—not a bad thing at a time when research funding from government and industry is drying up. If it works, personalized medicine promises a new age, a profound transition in the ways in which the healthcare system is structured, doctors are educated and patients are treated.

I am not a doctor, but I have written four books about the medical world and edited six anthologies comprising essays by doctors, patients, nurses and social workers. Few of the people about whom I have written or the authors with whom I have worked are happy or satisfied with the current American healthcare system. And why should they—or any of us—be satisfied? In our current system, million-dollar surgeries that are supposed to prolong life often don't work; needy children and their parents cry in anguish, waiting, unattended, in hospital emergency rooms for hours on end; patients in whom many resources have been invested do not modify their lifestyles or follow doctors' recommendations; and doctors can spare only an average of twelve minutes to listen to each patient's concerns, address complaints and prescribe a therapy. My interest in writing this book is grounded in a belief that personalized medicine promises an alternative—a way to make a significant and useful change for everyone. I am cautiously hopeful that it will lead to a positive transformation in the system, and subsequently to more affordable and better patient outcomes.

Brody's third scenario presents a childless couple who desperately want to start a family. But the man's genes show a strong susceptibility to the breast cancer (*BRCA*) gene. There's a 50% chance that he will pass on the mutation to his offspring. This doesn't mean that the child will inevitably develop breast cancer, but his or her risk will be significantly increased. And the child may also become a carrier.

The prospective parents choose in vitro fertilization. But before the fertilized eggs are implanted, the couple goes to a lab, where they have cells from the embryos sequenced. They ask the doctors to identify the embryos that don't carry the breast cancer mutation, and to implant only those embryos into the woman. The child is born free of breast cancer susceptibility—or at least, substantially so. Success story number three.

After Brody presents the three cases, he poses the million-dollar question to his audience, made up mostly of students and faculty from the University of Maryland, Baltimore County: while all of these ideas may eventually become reality, which are possible and happening today? The collective wish, of course, is that they all would be doable now—and the fear is that none of the ideas will ever be realized. After all, a half century ago, scientists were assuring us that the cure for cancer was just around the corner, and that hasn't exactly happened yet.

A few members of the audience hazard mumbled guesses, but they are in the dark. Even those who are well informed understand that the state of science changes by the day. Medications are concocted, procedures developed and tested. The floodgate is about to burst. Or so some scientists say.

Based on my recent experience talking to scientists, doctors and others, I am thinking that the first example is quite possible. I know that lots of interesting work is being done with the tailoring of medications to target tumors, and I have heard some amazing success stories. I think that the prostate cancer scenario could happen now—or at least in the very near future.

The second example is more complicated. There are genes and variants that indicate addictive personalities, but I'm pretty sure they aren't very conclusive or predictive. And what of the ethical and legal issues related to sequencing a ten-year-old's genome and sharing information related to the possibility of lung cancer and possible addictions with dozens—or more—people? And yet, technically speaking, this could happen now, as well, I think. It probably shouldn't happen—but it could.

The third scenario seems perhaps too sophisticated and advanced for the state of the art in personalized medicine, even though breast cancer is the primary area in which geneticists have made significant strides in applying personalized medicine procedures. This process of separating the good stuff from the bad stuff in a developing embryo is a wonderful idea—though possibly ethically complicated, depending how one defines "good stuff" and "bad stuff"—but it seems unlikely it's happening today.

Brody pauses only momentarily to sip from his paper cup before supplying the answer. Turns out I am wrong—at least, mostly. But new advances are occurring so quickly that, between the time Brody gave this talk, in October 2011, and the time you're reading this book, the first scenario he described may be possible. In 2011, we were not yet fully able to differentiate between dangerous and not-so-dangerous tumors in the prostate (or most anywhere else) and wipe them out so easily with drugs. But researchers at Memorial Sloan-Kettering Cancer Center have identified genetic subtypes of prostate cancer and can now predict, based on the subtype, whether a tumor is low or high risk. They have also developed nomograms for prostate cancer, graphs that help predict the best treatment for individual patients, based on a number of variables.

As for the second scenario, the addictive genes that the ten-year-old has are far less precisely predictive than would lead any physician to take such drastic actions on behalf of a patient, even if they were allowed—which they wouldn't be under today's privacy laws and probably never will be. Such information about a patient, even if available to doctors, could not be shared with teachers and guidance counselors.

But the third scenario, in which non-*BRCA*-carrying embryos are selected and implanted during in vitro fertilization, involves a procedure that is already being done successfully. It is called PGD—pre-implantation genetic diagnosis. Quite amazing.

Together, these three scenarios are a good, if partial, representation of the current state of personalized medicine and genetics. Scenarios one and two are "futuristic," as Brody would put it, but within our reach, maybe within the next ten years—though of course being "in reach" is far different from being put into practice. Even today there are many simple, proven genetic tests that could save many thousands of lives and prevent injuries and mistakes but are being ignored or delayed, mostly because of intransigent people, unwieldy systems and unprofitable bottom lines.

PGD, the procedure described in scenario three, for example, is obviously expensive, and not covered by healthcare insurance. Most doctors not only don't provide the service, they probably know very little about it, if they've heard of it at all. Almost inevitably, the result is that the privileged members of society have access to personalized therapies that are not available to everyone. This is a general overall objection from public health officials concerned with population-based medicine. A therapy may help a few people—but so much more may be accomplished by using the investment in dollars and effort to benefit society as a whole.

Of course, even once a procedure is scientifically feasible, there's usually a long way to go before it's integrated into society and the healthcare system, even if it only benefits a few. There's a huge gap to be bridged between cutting-edge medicine and the average general practice physician—and that's only one of the hurdles personalized medicine faces. Then there are the insurance companies and pharmaceutical corporations, which can be valuable partners or formidable obstacles—or both. Finally, the federal government and all of its many agencies and legislative branches, like the Federal Drug Administration (FDA), must buy in. The NIH, where Brody works, is pro-genetics, but it is a research institution—not a policymaking body. Ultimately, the challenge for the future will come down to the bottom line, to profit and loss: the economics must make sense to all parties involved. As you might imagine, none of this is happening very quickly.

And so it is difficult to predict with any certainty when enough parts of the personalized medicine puzzle will fall into place to really bring change to the healthcare system. A majority of scientists seem to agree that the slow transition is necessary—the science isn't actually there yet—but that the introduction of genetic analysis will be essential and inevitable. Just as embryos can be screened for genetic mutations, dozens of similarly amazing medical applications will be achieved someday. According to the scientists I have talked with, "someday" may mean ten years—or in another lifetime. There's a danger, after all, in assuming too much too quickly or hoping for miracles that are beyond our reach.

Meanwhile, however, there are already many ways we can utilize and benefit from the advances made to this point in genetics and personalized medicine. Patients and doctors need not be in limbo, waiting for the revolution to trickle down to them through government and industry. I hope that readers of this book will understand the importance of using the knowledge that we have amassed so far and of being proactive—taking advantage of what we are learning from science while pressuring our physicians, our government and our business leaders to learn along with us, while realizing that hard sacrifices and choices may be necessary to create meaningful change. It is equally critical that we remain cognizant and wary of where the personalized medicine revolution might lead—and of the principles and privileges we are potentially surrendering for the sake of longer life through genetics.

Screening out the fool's gold and shaping our healthcare El Dorado will, I believe, be our society's next and most vital challenge—a task even greater and more awesome than the sequencing of the human genome, which occurred a little more than a decade ago and precipitated the personalized medicine revolution. At the time, of course, the celebration of the translation of "the Book of Life" was an event that reverberated around the world.

PREFACE:
THE BIG EVENT

Picture the scene: June 26, 2000. The East Room of the White House is crowded with middle-aged men in suits and women in business attire, prominent members of the scientific community and members of Congress. At the front of the room is a podium with a gold presidential seal, flanked on both sides by large television monitors, behind which a long corridor with chandeliers and a row of thick white pillars leads to a set of double doors. The crowd, buzzing with conversation and expectation for what is about to be announced, quickly quiets when the double doors open and "Hail to the Chief" begins to play.

And then the tall, distinctive figure of the president of the United States, Bill Clinton, emerges and begins walking down the red-carpeted corridor toward the podium, accompanied by two men. On his left walks a tall, slender man with wire-rimmed glasses, slightly protruding ears, a neatly trimmed mustache and a friendly smile. This is Francis Collins, MD and PhD, director of the National Human Genome Research Institute (NHGRI), which was responsible for the federal government–supported Human Genome Project (HGP). Before taking over the HGP, Collins had been a geneticist at the University of Michigan, where he isolated genes responsible for cystic fibrosis, neurofibromatosis and Huntington's disease.

For a scientist, Collins is a bit of an anomaly. He commutes to work on a Harley-Davidson and frequently shoulders a guitar—he will play and sing sometimes very silly songs composed for different "formal" occasions—and he's got an unusual hairstyle, described by one observer as "an early Beatles mop top." He's a born-again Christian, the author of a best-selling book, *The Language of God: A Scientist Presents Evidence for Belief*, about his conversion to Christianity from atheism. The book argues that belief in a personal god—and the possibility of an occasional miracle—can coexist with belief in evolution:

"Science is not threatened by God; it is enhanced," Collins has written, and "God is most certainly not threatened by science; He made it all possible."

The man to the president's right, however—a shorter, chunkier fellow with a glittering, bald dome, red tie and wire glasses—might say that he himself, and not God, was the single most prominent contributor to the HGP. This is biologist J. Craig Venter, PhD, who has been described in numerous media outlets as a "man of supreme immodesty." Venter once asked a reporter, "Is my science of the level consistent with other people who have gotten the Nobel?" He answered the question himself: "Yes."

Collins and Venter are an unlikely pairing, but they have come together because they are most responsible for the work being celebrated today. Thankfully, however, they are separated by Clinton, who is well aware, as is most everyone in the audience, that the men are angry adversaries, embroiled in one of the most bitter and public disputes in the history of modern science.

The president pauses at the podium as Collins and Venter take their seats behind him. He waits for the welcoming applause to subside and then begins his remarks by describing another event that took place in this very spot nearly two centuries earlier, when President Thomas Jefferson and a trusted aide, Meriwether Lewis, spread out a "magnificent map . . . the product of his courageous expedition across the American frontier . . . a map that defined the contours and forever expanded the frontiers of our continent and our imagination."

Today, President Clinton said, the world "is joining us to behold a map of even greater significance." We are here, he said, to celebrate the completion of the first survey of the entire human genome—"Without a doubt . . . the most important, most wondrous map ever produced by mankind." Clinton was referring to the sequencing of the genetic code of human beings—what he and so many scientists were calling the Book of Life—the end of a process that began in 1983 and cost the federal government $3 billion to complete.

The word "genetics" comes from the Greek genetikos, which is linked to the word "genesis," as in the Bible, meaning origin. Genetics is anchored in DNA, deoxyribonucleic acid, the hereditary material that can be found in nearly every living cell. The information in DNA is stored as a code made up of four chemical bases: adenine (A), guanine (G), cytosine (C) and thymine (T). When people talk about sequencing the genome they are referring, essentially, to figuring out the order of humans' genetic material from beginning to end and decoding it, translating what looks like gobbledeygook into useful information that will potentially save lives and change the entire scope of how medicine is practiced and scientific research is performed.

To put this accomplishment into perspective, human DNA consists of 3.1 billion base pairs in each cell, a big number to begin with. But the overall extent of the cells—what they might mean as a mass—is nearly impossible to contemplate. And if you consider that two human beings each contribute twenty-three different chromosomes, made up of coils of DNA, to the creation of each new human being, then the potential combinations are beyond mind-boggling. The genetic code, which is what the president was talking about, is the set of rules that explains how DNA is translated into proteins. Among their many functions, proteins help the body's tissues and organs to function. Proteins give shape to cells and transport them through the body. Proteins can recognize and frequently protect the body from foreign or dangerous molecules.

In the audience that day was James D. Watson, who, not quite half a century earlier, as a brash young American scientist, had teamed with an Englishman named Francis Crick to discover the elegant structure of our genetic code. Clinton paused in his talk to address Watson directly and quip that the way Watson announced his discovery in the journal *Nature* was "one of the great understatements of all time." Clinton read from his teleprompter: "This structure [the double helix] has novel features, which are of considerable biological interest." The audience laughed, and Clinton said to Watson, "Thank you, sir."

It is unfortunate that another modest person—an Austrian friar—could not join Watson, Venter and Collins that day, because it is upon his shoulders perhaps more than on anyone else's that the entire genetics world stood in order to make the sequencing leap. In the middle of the nineteenth century, Gregor Mendel conducted breeding experiments with peas from his garden and became the first person to trace the characteristics of successive generations of a living thing. His work eventually led to the recognition of the basic laws of heredity—known as "Mendelian genetics." Traits or genetic inheritance, Mendel demonstrated, can be "dominant," which means that a gene is automatically passed on to another generation, or "recessive," meaning traits appear in one generation but may be missing in the next. The combinations of dominant and recessive genes determine eye color, hair type and whether ear wax will be wet or dry, but also, much more seriously, diseases people may have, in particular, rare single mutation or "monogenic" disorders, caused by a mutation—a change or alteration in a DNA sequence—that is passed from parent to offspring.

Clinton himself could not be singled out for understatement. To the contrary, he matched the mood of the moment by waxing eloquent. He invoked Galileo, who, when he "discovered he could use the tools of mathematics and mechanics to understand the motion of celestial bodies . . . felt, in the words of one eminent researcher, 'that he had learned the language in which God created the universe.' Today," said Clinton, "we are learning the language in which God created life."

In the coming years, Clinton continued, "doctors increasingly will be able to cure diseases like Alzheimer's, Parkinson's, diabetes and cancer by attacking their genetic roots . . . In fact, it is now conceivable that our children's children will know the term 'cancer' only as a constellation of stars." A few minutes later, he told British Prime Minister Tony Blair, appearing on the television monitors to deliver his own message from London about Britain's participation in the event, that his newborn son's life expectancy had "just gone up by about twenty-five years." In summation, Clinton proclaimed, "We are gaining ever more awe for the complexity, the beauty, the wonder of God's most divine and sacred gift. With this profound new knowledge, humankind is on the verge of gaining immense new power to heal." Clinton was in essence predicting a transformation—a new era of medicine of which the world had heretofore not conceived.

The statements from the two men flanking Clinton were equally profound. Francis Collins introduced a personal note, discussing his "beloved sister-in-law," a wonderful marionette artist who brought magic and joy to thousands of children with her art, and who died much too soon of breast cancer. "The hope and promise of understanding all of the genes in the genome and applying this knowledge to the development of powerful new tools came just too late for her."

Indeed, breast cancer victims, as President Clinton had pointed out in his talk, were already being treated successfully in clinical trials with sophisticated new drugs that precisely target the faulty genes and cancer cells, with little or no risk to healthy cells. This kind of successful treatment was the vision, the hope and the goal of the science that would soon come to be known as personalized medicine.

Craig Venter had actually been part of Collins's constituency and a beneficiary of federal financing, but one day in 1998, Venter approached Collins and told him that he was forming his own private company, Celera Genomics, to decode the genome on his own—and that he would finish the job in three years or less! Up to that point in time, the HGP had been bumbling along, aiming for a target ending date of 2005, a fact that may well have frustrated Venter, who often chose speed above practicality. "Craig likes to do high dives into empty pools," a former teacher once commented. "He tries to time it so the water is there before he hits the bottom."

Collins was at first merely annoyed at Venter for his sudden desertion, but his annoyance turned to fury after Venter calmly assured Collins that he was not trying to make him look bad. The field was wide open, and there were plenty of mammals to sequence. Celera would sequence the human genome, said Venter, and "you can do mouse." One can only imagine the anger Francis Collins must have felt at Venter's arrogance and his ambush—not to mention the feelings of vulnerability. After all, the success of the HGP was intimately and intricately entwined with Collins's reputation. If the HGP was perceived to be a success, then Collins, more than any other single individual, would be the beneficiary, at least professionally. His reputation would suffer significantly if Venter, the arrogant upstart, trumped him and the HGP. Venter was also profit motivated. While Collins and others envisioned any potential financial profits emanating from genetic sequencing going toward the public good, Venter wanted to make gobs of money (albeit to support further research, but in the private sector).

The for-profit group Venter formed and led at Celera had, among other achievements, adopted what was called "shotgun sequencing"—a shortcut technique that contrasted with the slow, methodical "scientific" way in which the HGP group was working under Collins. Eventually, "shot-gunning" proved to do the job faster and more or less just as well, however, and Collins's group adopted it, if reluctantly.

At that point, Collins realized that he did not want to come in second—especially to Venter—and so he agreed to a compromise (if not a truce) in order not to take a back seat to Celera. Thus the announcement was made in the year 2000 with both groups getting equal credit—though technically, this was just a "working draft" of the genome, and the complete genome wasn't sequenced by HGP until 2003.

It was actually President Clinton who had pressured the two scientists to put aside their resentments and appear together. At the time, Clinton's second term was nearly complete; he had been embarrassed by the Monica Lewinsky scandal, and was working full-blast to spotlight the positive accomplishments of his administration, even though he had inherited the HGP from the Reagan era. Clinton had forced the issue. He had asked his science adviser, Neal Lane, to "Fix it . . . make these guys work together." And so in early May, meeting at a mutual friend's house and talking over pizza and beer, the two worked out their differences. Later, the friend observed, "I don't think I've ever seen them as tense as they were that day."

Collins was not the only scientist under pressure. Venter's tactless egocentricity had diminished his reputation, and when, in March 2000, Clinton and Prime Minister Blair announced that all genomic information should be free to the public, the value of Celera stock fell by 19%.

In contrast to his braggadocio, Venter's presentation was underwhelming. Since he was shorter than the two men who preceded him, he first fumbled around with a standing stool to reach the podium and microphones. His bald dome shined in the bright lights, and he delivered his remarks in a numbing monotone; he was so plain and ordinary looking he could have passed for an IRS auditor, reading a long list of numbers without emotion or inflection. His wire glasses slid down to the bridge of his nose while he read.

The substance of his remarks, however, was provocative. Celera, Venter explained, had independently sequenced the genome of five individuals: two males and three females, of Asian, Caucasian, Hispanic and African-American ancestry. In the five genomes, he announced, "there is no way to tell one ethnicity from another."

Later, he said, "One of the wonderful discoveries that my colleagues and I have made while decoding the DNA of over two dozen species, from viruses to bacteria to plants to insects, and now human beings, is that we're all connected to the commonality of the genetic code in evolution. When life is reduced to its very essence, we find that we have many genes in common with every species on earth, and that we're not so different from one another. You may be surprised to learn that your sequencers are greater than 90% identical to proteins in other animals." This was an important message, though difficult for many Americans to accept then and even now: that all people of various colors and physical characteristics are more or less biologically identical. The differences between races are negligible.

And while this was a grand event signifying a momentous scientific milestone, Venter pointed out that the world at large—the potential patients this potential new power to heal might serve—weren't impressed with the sequencing achievement or optimistic about its positive impact. Results of a CNN-Time poll released that very day, he said, revealed that 46% of all Americans polled believed that the impact of the HGP would be negative. Many believed that the sequencing of the human genome would diminish humanity and take the mystery out of life.

Venter—and CNN—were foreshadowing an issue that now is becoming increasingly relevant and evident. Taking a person apart genetically can seem unnecessarily and overwhelmingly revealing, like undressing them in a public place and in a very intimate way—to their core. Think of it. Even though we live in our bodies, we know very little about the substance of the materials from which we were made or the ancient secrets they might reveal. For good or bad, genetics says something very fundamental about who we are or are not.

And the more we learn about biology and heredity, the more cautious many people are becoming about sharing that information—for a variety of reasons. Most people I have talked with are wary of the ramifications of sharing what can be learned from their DNA with others. In their remarks, Collins, Venter and Clinton all referred to the protections that would be essential in this new genetically personalized world. President Clinton said, "As we unlock the secrets of the human genome, we must work simultaneously to ensure that new discoveries never pry open the doors of privacy. And we must guarantee that genetic information cannot be used to stigmatize or discriminate against any individual or group."

Venter's remarks, like those of Collins, also contained a personal element: "Thirty-three years ago, as a young man serving in the medical corps in Vietnam," he said, "I learned firsthand how tenuous our hold on life can be. That experience inspired my interest in learning how the trillions of cells in our bodies interact to create and sustain life. When I witnessed firsthand that some men live through devastating trauma to their bodies, while others died after giving up from seemingly small wounds, I realized that the human spirit was at least as important as our physiology." Today, studies point to the fact that psychological characteristics of the human personality and spirit may also be genetically influenced.

The ceremony lasted only forty-one minutes. But it inspired high hopes for the future of medicine across the world. Optimism in that room was boundless. "There is no other scientific enterprise that humankind has mounted in an organized way that compares to this," Collins had recently told Congress. "I am sure that history will look back at this in a hundred years and say, 'This was the most significant thing that humankind has tried to do, scientifically.'"

In other recent venues, Collins was more effusive than even Clinton had been at the White House. In ten years, he predicted, we should expect widely available genetic tests to determine predispositions to more than a dozen major causes of illness and death, including genetic tests to pinpoint smokers at high risk for lung cancer, genetic tests to identify men in whom prostate cancer will spread most quickly, genetic tests to predict heart disease and isolate those most susceptible, genetic tests to identify those in a high-risk category for diabetes. By 2020, Collins predicted, physicians will have many new drugs to work with, tailored to an individual's genetic make-up, and will be able to pinpoint methods to determine dosage. By 2030, he said, "I predict that comprehensive, genomics-based healthcare will become the norm, with individualized preventive medicine and early detection of illnesses by molecular surveillance; gene therapy and gene-based therapy will be available for many diseases." Later, he observed that genetics and personalized medicine represented the "greatest revolution since Leonardo."

Collins was imagining a world in which science—specifically the HGP—would not only impact society globally, but would make an extraordinary difference on a very individual basis. Knowing so much more about our genetic make-up and the effects of our heritage—our future fates!—we would be more likely to change our behaviors, to exercise regularly, to eat more healthily, to stop smoking, to minimize alcohol intake.

In other words, this great burst of knowledge would lead to patient empowerment and self-awareness. Resources would be targeted to prevention rather than treatment. Doctors, general practitioners, would be less encumbered because people would be doctoring themselves and consequently minimizing ordinary ailments. This was the world that Collins and many of his colleagues predicted, and the scientific community was not alone in its effusiveness. Even before the sequencing of the genome was complete, members of the media were riding the HGP bandwagon. Take, for example, this cover story in *Time Magazine*: "Genetics: The Future Is Now." The publication date preceded the White House announcement by a half-dozen years: January 17, 1994. *Time's* editors were way ahead of even the most optimistic of the scientists.

This, then, was the mood of the majority of the men and women in science and the media a little more than a decade ago—full speed ahead because with this announcement a new era was practically upon us. We were at the cusp of a revolution which would bring nothing less than medical miracles.

This optimism from the experts and the media reminds me of the mood of the country at the dawning of the space age. In 1969, the entire world was captivated by the astronaut Neil Armstrong taking his "one small step for man, one giant leap for mankind" on the moon, and scientists, engineers and world leaders predicted a revolution in technology along with a vast exploration of many new worlds.

Now, the sequencing of the genome promises to help us "boldly go where no man has gone before," as *Star Trek*'s Captain James T. Kirk would put it—but on earth, through medicine. It is easy to fantasize: Someday genetic sequencing will be instantaneous—and inexpensive. Diagnosis for all diseases will be achieved through a universal blood test. A silver-bullet pill or an injection of genetic elixir will kill cancerous tumors. Diabetes and other chronic diseases will be eradicated.

At the White House a dozen years ago, President Clinton declared that we were approaching an era in which doctors would be endowed with an "immense new power to heal." How close we are to that era (or how far away we remain from achieving those dreams and ambitions and bringing the science to patients—real people and not just mice and test tubes—in the hospital or in the doctor's office, where personalized medicine must begin) probably can't be determined accurately just yet.

What has already been determined, however, by the work of genetics pioneers like Collins, Venter and the physicians and patients who have followed in their footsteps, is that the emergence of such an era is in process, and inevitable. And considering today's broken healthcare system, the changes promised by personalized medicine can come not a moment too soon.

CHAPTER 1:
THE CANCER
DOCTORS FEAR MOST

In December 2009, nearly a decade after the White House ceremony marking the sequencing of the genome, Michael Saks waited in a neat, orderly office on the sprawling campus of the Mayo Clinic in Scottsdale, Arizona, to meet with a genetic counselor and learn the results of a blood test. Several weeks earlier, he had taken a test, which, by detecting mutations in the *BRCA1* and *BRCA2* genes, assesses an individual's risk of developing hereditary breast or ovarian cancer. His test was done by Myriad Genetics, which does all genetic analysis for *BRCA1* and *BRCA2*.

Saks knew that the results of the blood test might provide interesting information, but he was also aware that it would not help determine to any great degree whether he is especially vulnerable to the disease he fears most: pancreatic cancer. *BRCA* mutations do increase the risk of pancreatic cancer, but they are not nearly as predictive for that disease as they are for breast cancer.

The risk of getting pancreatic cancer has haunted Michael Saks for most of his life. His mother had pancreatic cancer. He watched her die—she died quickly, within a year-—as he cared for her, and the memory of her suffering profoundly affected him, because he knew that pancreatic cancer could be hereditary and that his mother's fate could be his own.

In August 2011, Steve Jobs, cofounder of Apple Inc., who battled pancreatic cancer for half a decade, resigned as the company's CEO. He died two months later. The news about Jobs and about pancreatic cancer, generally, is sobering for Saks or others in similar circumstances. Jobs survived longer than almost any pancreatic cancer victim. But the statistics are damning: Fewer than 5% of those diagnosed with pancreatic cancer are alive five years later. Pancreatic cancer is a silent enemy; it grows secretly, undetectable, for decades. When it is discovered it is almost always too late to take action: pancreatic cancer is usually discovered only after it has spread to other organs.

Every day we read about incredible accomplishments in the world of medicine—from face transplants to robotic surgery—as well as the miracle of DNA. And yet, scientists and physicians seem to be powerless to stop certain diseases. Dr. Mehmet Oz, the popular TV physician, once did a segment on his daily TV show called "The Cancer Doctors Fear Most." It was about pancreatic cancer.

Saks is short and balding, with wire-rimmed eyeglasses and a salt-and-pepper beard, haphazardly trimmed. He speaks with a careful thoughtfulness, grinding out his answers to questions and observations about his life and fate with a somewhat flat affect and a persistent precision. A law professor and a social psychologist who works with lawyers and judges to foster an appreciation of the usefulness of scientific experiments and studies, he invariably pauses before responding to questions, almost as if he is measuring his interactions in court in front of a judge. He replies only after he reviews what he is going to say in his mind, a process that takes a few long seconds.

Saks was living in Boston, a young professor climbing the tenure ladder at Boston College, at the time his mother was first diagnosed. But he had been visiting home on the day when his mother returned from the doctor's office and shared her news. She said: "I have a year to live."

The doctors hadn't pronounced her death sentence, Saks remembers. The doctors were characteristically noncommittal. But his mother knew. In the 1950s, Saks's paternal grandmother had died of pancreatic cancer, and so his mother had witnessed firsthand the way in which pancreatic cancer can devastate a seemingly healthy human being in a relative instant.

Even now, many years later, Saks's flashing memories of his grandmother's demise are sometimes vivid: "I was five or six years old, and I had this awareness of voices," he says. "'Grandmother is very ill—Grandmother is very ill. She is going to the hospital. They have done some exploratory surgery. They took a look. They said, 'Oh, oh, there is nothing we can do. Just close her up, so she'll die.' And she did."

His mother's diagnosis was devastating to Saks—and sobering. Not only was he losing a parent. But his mother's cancer, especially when combined with the identical diagnosis on the other side of the family, could also foreshadow the possibility of his own doom.

At first, Saks wanted to help his mother fight her disease. He is the kind of person who, faced with a problem, takes action. He looked into many alternative therapies, including macrobiotic diets and mental imaging, but the writing was on the wall. In the early 1980s, the survival rate for pancreatic cancer was 2%. It is not much better today. Pancreatic cancer is the fourth leading cause of death in this country from cancer. An estimated 40,000 Americans died in 2010 from pancreatic cancer.

Michael Saks's two siblings, a brother and sister, were unable to care for their mother on a regular basis. Saks resigned himself to helping his mother in any way possible, knowing that she would not be alive too much longer. He found himself on a plane every other weekend, heading home to do whatever was needed, which, it turned out, was to try to help his mother deal with the pain—or, more precisely, deal with the doctors who administered the pain medication. His mother had decided that she did not want to try to fight any longer, even though the doctors were campaigning for a final desperate intervention: surgery. But surgery for pancreatic cancer is pretty awful, Saks says: "They cut you open and take everything out, put some of it back in, and nothing ever works the same again." Saks was right: surgery was hardly a viable option, especially at that time. Even now, it may gain months of survival—but not a lot more. Steve Jobs, with all his resources, was able to have an expensive liver transplant—but he too succumbed.

Frustrated and in constant agony, Saks's mother asked her son to telephone her oncologist and explain that she was not looking for a miracle: all she wanted was some short-term relief. Saks, she assumed, would speak the doctors' language; after all, he was an educated man, a PhD psychologist in a law school who taught judges how to make more accurate and informed decisions, among other things, while she was just a housewife. The doctors might not listen to her, but her son the doctor-professor could make them understand her needs. Saks telephoned the oncologist and explained the situation. "And the doctor gave me a bad time," Saks remembers. "He said, quite bluntly, 'Don't you care if your mother lives or dies?'"

Doctors were confident that they knew what was right for their patients back then. In the 1980s, we were still ensconced in the era of doctor paternalism—doctors were a priesthood, likened to deities. They could do no wrong—and medical school was a nearly guaranteed path to prestige, influence and money. As many physicians, young and old, will attest, the situation has gradually changed over the past two decades, although maybe not substantially enough. The cost of technology—and perhaps the overuse of technology in fear of being accused of malpractice—is out of control. Establishing a private practice unencumbered by bottom-line pressures from insurance companies and behemoth medical centers is becoming increasingly difficult. But the arrogance that Saks experienced from his mother's doctors back then persists in certain milieus—and lingers vividly in Saks's memory. Decades later, he remains bitter.

"So I am supposed to feel guilty that the doctor wants to do what he wants to do and my mother won't let him?" Saks exclaims. "That wasn't right." His mother knew her fate and was trying to take control of her destiny, to the extent she could, Saks says. It was her prerogative. What ever happened to patient-driven healthcare, he wondered?

Personalized medicine advocates will tell you today that this is exactly the goal of personalized medicine—focusing first and foremost on the patient, and not on the system that supports the patient (and the physician). Of course, most doctors will insist that this has always been the goal of their practice, which may be true, although perhaps not a reality, at least not as often as they wish.

At the time he took the Myriad test, Michael Saks was healthy, physically fit and professionally productive; he was, at 63, near the same age as his mother when she died. "I have relatives on both sides of the family who have died of pancreatic cancer," says Saks. And then he pauses and lowers his voice. Despite his prestige, experience and education, this is clearly a worry plaguing him. Finally he says: "And so might I." In reality, only 10% of pancreatic cancer victims have a family history of the disease—and yet the knowledge produced in him a haunting, ever-present anxiety.

It wasn't only the perceived hereditary curse that made Michael Saks so unsettled—it was the prospect of dealing with the unwieldy medical system that makes sickness or even the threat of being sick and hospitalized so uncomfortable and frustrating. During the many times I talked with him, he was attempting to help his sister, who is somewhat handicapped, be admitted for a procedure and subsequently rehabilitated and discharged from the hospital, and he was experiencing the frustration of fighting a system that relies on decisions made by various physicians who do not communicate and administrators who follow regulations that may make sense for the "universal" patient but often ignore individuals' needs. Hospitals should be healing institutions and not necessary evils, places to be avoided because they are so unpleasant.

And then there was the mystery of not knowing whether the cancer is welling up inside you. Saks returned to ponder this mystery repeatedly. When such a worry is on your mind, every ache and pain can be exacerbated; you can close your eyes and imagine the cancer growing inside of you, like worms eating away at your insides, while you are helplessly unaware.

There are, currently, no real diagnostic tools to detect pancreatic cancer. There are only three early-detection tests that have been shown to prevent cancer deaths: mammogram, Pap smear and colonoscopy. There are other early detection tests—including screens for prostate cancer and melanoma—but these have not been shown to extend life span in patients. In some cases, such tests can even increase patient mortality by leading to unnecessary intervention. In other words, even if someone devised an early-detection test for pancreatic cancer, there's no guarantee it would extend anyone's life. Pancreatic cancer is like a time bomb: by the time you know enough to take action it is much too late, as Saks's mother had discovered. All you can do is worry, wonder and wait. At least that is what Michael Saks had always assumed.

In 2009, Saks was living in Tempe/Phoenix and was regents professor of law and psychology in the Center for Law, Science & Innovation at the Sandra Day O'Connor Law School at Arizona State University (ASU). The president of ASU asked him to give a talk to a select group of community leaders and potential contributors, as part of a series of talks offered on a regular basis, and invited him to attend the talk scheduled for the month before his presentation so that he could get the feel of what he was being asked to do.

The talk Saks attended was given by a professor in ASU's Biodesign Institute, who, in his remarks, mentioned research that could someday lead to methods for isolating the genes that cause pancreatic cancer and developing interventions to mute them. This was interesting information: drugs might be able to eliminate the necessity of surgery. Or—even better—drugs might be able to wipe out the effects of the gene.

The professor delivering the talk was not an oncologist, and his remarks about pancreatic cancer were only tangentially related to his topic. But they held special interest for Saks, in the audience, who suddenly realized that there might be actions he could take besides sitting around and worrying.

This was the first time Saks had heard the term "personalized medicine." Scientists at ASU and at medical centers across the country, he learned, were working with researchers at Translational Genomics Research Institute (TGen) and the Mayo Clinic in Scottsdale, a few miles down the road from campus. Translational research means the process of translating basic scientific discoveries into clinical applications—building a bridge between lab-bench discoveries and the patient at bedside. Saks decided that if there were things he could do, then he wanted to find out about them now.

The medical world has long held patients hostage. From hour-long delays in waiting rooms to withholding information or explanations from helpless and unknowing patients, the doctor has had steadfast control. And even though you have the perfect right to read your medical chart or retain copies of your medical records, it is nearly impossible to do this without a fight—or without jumping through many unnecessary hoops. And while it is true that patients often do not listen to their doctors' best advice, it is also true that information can be empowering to patients and lead them into positive action, in the same way the professor's lecture led Saks to take action.

More and more, patients are asking questions and finding answers that their physicians previously could not or would not provide. The search for genetic links to disease is, in essence, a search for information—and this search is increasingly carried out by all of the actors in the process, from scientists and physicians to patients and their families. True personalized medicine is an action-oriented team effort, and the team includes an obvious yet heretofore unacknowledged member: the patient.

"As a psychologist with a focus on human behavior," says Saks, "my inclination is to want to act, to problem-solve and not just worry. I was 63 and the next year I would be 64, my mother's age at her death, so I will probably get very nervous on my birthday, which is kind of dumb, because your cells are not on an exact timetable. And my mother was different than me in many ways—her diet, her environment. She lived in Philadelphia and I was in the desert." But he needed to know—or he *thought* he needed to know—everything he could learn about the disease that threatened him.

Saks had once waxed philosophical about the mystery of knowing—or not knowing—what a person wants to know about his or her own health. It is a very personal and very convoluted way of thinking and reasoning—or, as the case may be, not reasoning. "Maybe I only want to know a few things about my health and well-being and then stop before it gets to the point that I know too much," he mused. "Or maybe I don't want to know anything sometimes. Or maybe, other times, I want to know everything and do everything conceivable, no matter how miniscule. Maybe people go through all stages of knowing and wanting to know at different times, depending on mood and the information available to them at any given moment."

His point was that every patient is different, and every patient's feelings and predilections often swing radically, like a pendulum. Saks is a scientist, however, and, as such, he thought he needed to know everything about his own health, no matter how frightening or daunting. So despite the fact that—with regards to pancreatic cancer, at least—research into early detection and eventual intervention was in the earliest stages, Saks felt that he had a direction. He could take action, no matter how preliminary and inconclusive. This is a natural tendency that many people share: a belief that doing something is better than doing nothing. On the other hand, of course, there are many people who would choose not knowing and inaction over finding out something that they did not necessarily want to learn.

Saks learned that some of the pancreatic cancer research was being done at the Mayo Clinic at Scottsdale, so he moved his healthcare there. He found a suitable general practitioner at Mayo to give him his annual physicals and to involve him in a genetics-screening program. This was how he came to work with the genetic counselor he was waiting to meet: Katherine Hunt, the coordinator of Mayo's genetic counseling program. She began her work with Saks in the same way in which doctors have come to know their patients down through the ages: by taking a family history. In preparation for their first meeting, she asked Saks to gather as much information as possible about his family on both sides, so that she would be able to build a map of health issues that had manifested in the family, as a starting point. This is how personalized medicine begins.

CHAPTER 2:
CAN WE READ
THE BOOK OF LIFE?

As a patient, as most of us are from time to time, how should you expect to be treated by your doctors? Yes, of course, politely and efficiently: You want your doctors to respect your time and not force you to sit in a waiting room for an hour before they will see you. And you want their undivided attention once you are admitted to the inner sanctum of the examination room so that they can understand your health issues and help you—with medication, additional testing or referral, whatever is needed. Most of all, in the perfect world, you want your doctors to understand that you are unique, inside and outside, and not necessarily like everybody else. The medical center or doctor's office should not seem like a factory. The patient should not feel like a commodity on a conveyor belt. You are an individual—just like your doctor.

Obviously, a patient's experience differs with each doctor—some doctors are much more engaging and "people friendly" than others—but in fact most doctors do try to pay attention to who you are and how you are feeling; to respond to your symptoms and concerns when examining you, one-on-one; and to help you get well and stay well. That's their mission as doctors, an anchoring element of the Hippocratic Oath.

The basic idea behind personalized medicine is as old as the practice of medicine itself. Hippocrates proclaimed: "It is more important to know what sort of person has a disease than to know what sort of disease a person has." William Osler, considered to be the father of modern medicine, echoed Hippocrates more than two millennia later: "Care more particularly for the individual patient than for the special features of the disease."

But in practice, in the modern era, your doctors' decisions and actions related to diagnosis and treatment are more often than not homogenized—and not personalized. Here is what I mean:

Doctor practice and patient treatment have remained constant—you might even say stagnant—over the past century: doctors have treated patients based on the results of large epidemiological studies. If, say, most of 4,000 patients suffering from diabetes show significant improvement after receiving a certain drug, then physicians prescribe those drugs to patients with similar symptoms. This is why physicians read medical journals, where the results of such studies are published. The patient deserves to be treated with a proven therapy that works. And this process works—to a point.

But—and this is a big *but*—while the subjects in such studies are usually similar (e.g., all women, or all two-pack-a-day smokers), their individuality or differences have likely not been taken into account. Studies may narrow participants down by symptoms, age or other characteristics, but the people who have been studied remain generalized and categorized; who and what they are at a biological level, an environmental level and a behavioral level are often not primary factors that have been considered.

Personalized medicine, in contrast, means defining the person in as many ways as possible in order to more precisely pinpoint diagnosis and tailor treatment to each individual's needs. Personalized medicine intensifies the level of examination, leading to a more targeted treatment. It decreases the "hit or miss" or "trial and error" aspect inherent in medicine as practiced today. Dr. Aaron Chiechanover, who was awarded the Nobel Prize in Chemistry in 2004 for his discovery of how cells reduce unwanted proteins, describes the type of medicine currently being practiced in the United States as "one size fits all—much like a pajama, uniform and supposedly applicable to everyone." Personalized medicine, however, is like a suit "sitting right on the shoulders, button down . . . like it is tailored for us." Scientists and pharmacologists refer to this tailoring or targeting of medication, which is one significant aspect of personalized medicine, as "pharmacogenomics."

A good example of pharmacogenomics is the application of warfarin, the most commonly prescribed blood thinner in North America. Also known by the brand name Coumadin, this is an effective and relatively safe drug that has been widely used since the 1950s, when it was used to treat President Eisenhower after a heart attack. And yet, determining the best dose of warfarin for an individual patient can be difficult—and dangerous. If the dose is too high, patients can suffer from internal bleeding; too low, and they are vulnerable to stroke from blood clots. So doctors do their best to find the sweet spot for each patient; they prescribe a dose, do some tests, adjust the dose and so on. Ideally, they find the appropriate recipe for each patient.

Recently scientists have discovered that certain genetic variations in patients have a significant impact on the effectiveness of warfarin. Studies indicate that integrating genetic testing with warfarin therapy—that is, screening patients before prescribing an initial dose of the drug—could prevent as many as 85,000 serious bleeding events and 17,000 strokes annually, in the process saving United States taxpayers more than $1 billion, according to a working paper published several years ago by the AEI-Brookings Joint Center for Regulatory Studies. Warfarin is only one example, of course; similar studies confirm the effectiveness of genetic testing for other blood thinners, including Plavix. All medicines would be targeted to the individual patient, if personalized medicine were to be practiced in the full-blown way. Doctors write nearly four billion prescriptions every year, and about two million of those prescriptions result in hospitalizations for adverse drug reactions. Conservative estimates suggest that somewhere between 60,000 and 80,000 of those patients will die, and the number may be as high as 100,000. Not all of these fatalities and hospitalizations relate to genetics, but testing can make a difference.

Another facet to the evolving field of personalized medicine is biomedical informatics: using computers to share information about patients, research and medications, in order to treat patients more effectively and efficiently. John Gennari of the University of Washington describes it as interdisciplinary, connecting "computer science, medicine, biology and healthcare, and [providing] a synergy that goes beyond anything that researchers in any single domain can provide." Consider, for a moment, the explosion of medical data available worldwide because of the sequencing of the genome; consider, too, the amount of information collected over the years by physicians and medical centers and written, mostly by hand, into patients' charts. The idea is to digitize and synthesize all this information so that scientists and physicians have available "the right information at the right time for the right treatment." Many medical schools are establishing biomedical informatics PhD programs to prepare information-age engineers for the personalized-medicine era, and at some schools medical students are required to take biomedical informatics courses so that they will know how to access the most definitive research.

A crucial aspect of personalized medicine—and perhaps its strongest attraction—is the shift from "reactive" to "preventive" medicine. Most adults don't see doctors until they have symptoms of disease—a rash, say, or an ongoing soreness or pain. Or people will wait for their annual physical to see a doctor—by which time it might be too late or considerably more complicated to treat the disease or symptom. Practicing personalized medicine, conducting family histories and utilizing genetic tests, may help doctors identify potential conditions before they become serious and harmful—or even predict them before they occur, when treatment is possible and relatively inexpensive.

The power of prediction is what Lawrence Brody was stressing to the students in his audience. It reminds me of the baseball book and movie *Moneyball*, which chronicled the Oakland A's general manager Billy Bean's efforts to carefully and intricately computerize and analyze the history and performance of every ball player on his team, as well as those for whom he traded, so that he could predict with relative certainty how they would play and what they could achieve on an individualized basis—and how they could become better and make fewer mistakes. His small-market, grossly underdog team won the American League championship that year.

Unfortunately, the A's lost the World Series, so Bean's system of analysis wasn't foolproof. This, too, parallels the inchoate state of personalized medicine, and the promise of future developments in medical research will likely lead us closer and closer to foolproof medical analysis. Prediction is an anchoring element of personalized medicine—leading to the possibility of early diagnosis and intervention or, better yet, prevention, stopping disease before it starts. This is at the root of the personalized medicine movement. But Billy Bean probably knows more about his ballplayers' potential ability to field and hit than their doctors know about their health and well-being. Conceivably, today Mr. Goodwrench knows more about your automobile after a state inspection and tune-up than your doctors know about your health on a regular basis.

Consider this: healthcare expenditures in the United States have quadrupled over the past two decades. By 2050, unless there are significant changes to the system, more than one third of our gross domestic product (GDP) will be devoted to healthcare. There are many reasons for this, including the fact that new interventions are considerably more expensive than earlier therapies and that there has been a disproportional emphasis on the development of drugs to treat and cure rather than on diagnostics and prevention. A focus on personalized medicine would lead to a more equitable balance. This makes sense: the sooner we know about a problem, the sooner we can try to address it. The sooner we resolve it (or, even better, prevent it), the more pain and suffering we avoid and the more resources we rescue. In 2009, according to CBS's *60 Minutes*, "Medicare paid $50 billion just for doctor and hospital bills in the last two months of patients' lives. That's more than the budget of the Department of Homeland Security or the Department of Education, and it has been estimated that 20 to 30% of these medical expenditures may have no meaningful impact." An emphasis on diagnosis and prevention could help lead to a shift in resources.

I once wrote a book about organ transplantation. For my research, I immersed myself in what was then the largest organ transplant center in the world. Over a period of four years, I lived, off and on, in a facility for patients (and families) who were waiting for organs to become available for transplant or who were recovering from transplant surgery. I had access to the transplant operating rooms, so I was able to observe surgeries—often ten to twelve hours long, and very bloody—for liver, heart and heart/lung transplants. Many of the patients I wrote about died either in surgery or in the weeks following, though twenty years later, a few are still alive.

In comparison to the roller-coaster path of personalized medicine, the path of making organ transplantation therapeutic was relatively straightforward and linear: surgeons perfected the surgical techniques one by one until every subtle step was choreographed and they had established a tried-and-true process. This didn't eliminate mistakes and failures or rule out new ideas and improvements, and the man or woman with the scalpel or cauterizing gun still had to think on his or her feet. After the surgery, the battle continued, as the immune system tried to reject the organ. Over time—months or even years—immunosuppressive medications that could control the immune system without harming the transplant recipient were developed and tested in clinical trials. In fact, this process of developing immunosuppressive medications turned out to be more challenging than the surgery itself. Eventually a breakthrough drug called cyclosporine was developed from a material extracted from an obscure fungus. That drug considerably improved organ transplantation recipient survival—and another drug, initially called FK-506 (now Tacrolimus), was eventually introduced that increased the immunosuppressive power and resilience even more safely and efficiently. Again, this was a linear process; one improvement followed another.

It was a harrowing time, when surgeons and immunologists were developing those procedures and medications, but organ transplantation became steadily more successful, to the point now that you can consider the surgery and the immunosuppressive regimen almost routine, if still dangerous. The more practical limitation on transplantation today is our society's inability to supply enough organs to meet the need of the population. The many artificial organ devices developed over the years have proved to be inadequate, and there are far more candidates on the organ-transplant list than there are available organs or people willing to donate.

If you consider that organ transplantation began in earnest in the mid to late 1950s, when the first series of successful kidney transplants occurred, then it is easy to say that the process from beginning to end took nearly three quarters of a century—and the process remains unfinished. Transplantation is still expensive and not without serious risk. And there are many roadblocks. For example, although we can transplant kidneys, hearts, lungs and livers, pancreatic transplantation remains unsuccessful—so much so that surgeons are no longer even attempting the procedure. Our ability to store organs—to keep them alive for long periods, waiting to match the best donor with the best recipient—is woefully inadequate. But the science is progressing. We are well past the early stages. And organ transplantation is only a very small aspect of the surgical world—a chapter, at most, in a textbook. And surgery itself is only one aspect of medicine.

But transplantation is relatively narrow in scope when compared with personalized medicine—a game-changing technology as potentially disruptive as the Internet has been. Personalized medicine represents an entirely new paradigm. When personalized medicine becomes a reality, even at the most elementary level, nearly every aspect of a doctor's approach to patient care and treatment will undergo a radical transformation. Nothing will be as we know it today.

Bruce R. Korf is the president for clinical genetics of the American College of Medical Genetics and the Sara Crews Finley professor of medical genetics and chair of the department of genetics at the University of Alabama, Birmingham. He sees the doctor's role changing rapidly in response to new developments. Doctors in the early days of the twentieth century, says Korf, "were like pilots flying a single-engine plane with an open cockpit and with only three dials to look at; you could get in trouble, but chances are you could figure out how to get out of trouble most of the time." Today, however, a pilot would be unable to land a 747 if all of the computers went out simultaneously, and doctors may soon be in a similar position: "You can't fly by the seat of your pants anymore because you don't have the capability of taking into account all of the thousands of variables that constitute a plane in its proper operation. There are too many moving parts to keep it all in your head."

The immensity of the challenge presented by the completion of the HGP was not initially expected by those scientists laboring away at the bench in the 1980s and 1990s. Before the HGP, it was commonly believed that humans were incredibly complicated creatures, with as many as 100,000 genes to recognize and map. But every year, as the pace of research accelerated and more data was collected, estimates of the number of genes in the human body, contrary to all expectations, decreased. By the time the sequencing of the genome was announced, the tally of human genes had dipped down to around 25,000. "It was a big blow to mankind and to my colleagues," one geneticist told me, "to realize that yeast has 6,000 genes. Onions have more genes than humans do."

The hope at the time was that the sequencing of the genome would simplify and improve the practice of medicine—perhaps not right away, but with the Book of Life open, we would learn to read from its pages and make definite connections between genetic mutations and disease, and then develop appropriate therapeutic agents, or drugs. The thought then was that many diseases were rooted in single mutations, the kind of monogenic disorders described by Mendel, the Austrian friar, in which a mutation passed from parent to offspring results in disease—the expression of the mutation. Huntington's disease is monogenic, as is cystic fibrosis.

Prior to the HGP, it was relatively easy for experienced doctors to identify known genetic abnormalities—for example, cleft lips, developmental delay, cystic fibrosis and phenylketonuria (PKU), a metabolic disease causing mental retardation and other neurological difficulties—by observation. Pediatrics became an anchoring area for genetics in the early 1960s, with the development of chromosome analysis to diagnose Down syndrome and, following soon thereafter, amniocentesis, a procedure performed during pregnancy in which amniotic fluid is withdrawn from a woman's uterus to test for problems, including genetic defects, in the fetus.

Newborn screening has since been expanded and is regulated on a state-by-state basis for as many as fifty disorders. These are mostly not very sexy or highly promoted diseases, but they can be deadly, like maple syrup urine disease, in which the body is unable to process certain protein building blocks (amino acids) properly. Children who suffer from this genetic recessive disease—that is, they have to receive the mutation from both parents—are at risk of becoming profoundly critically ill, and they smell just like maple syrup: sweet. A half-century ago, few of these children survived into adulthood, but now, with early intervention and careful monitoring, most are able to lead normal and healthy lives.

The hope was that the HGP would provide the keys to figuring out other, less straightforward diseases, and to make this *predictive, preventive* medicine work—practice this personalized medicine approach and philosophy—on a much larger, all-inclusive scale.

"We spent our time—the last 100 years," says Lawrence Brody, "tackling the Mendelian—or single-gene—challenges, but now we are trying to deal with those that are more complicated."

Even before the HGP was completed, scientists realized that not every disease would be simple to diagnose or cure and not all mutations would be monogenic. But most researchers assumed that there was more often than not a direct connection—a single gene or, at most, a very small cluster of genes—for each disease. Identify and obliterate the gene or cluster, and you would cure or eradicate the disease. That was the general scientific wisdom up until a decade ago, and scientists were certainly naively unaware of the complications they were about to confront. They did not conceive of how many hereditary disorders would turn out to be multi-factorial, meaning that they are caused by a combination of small variations in genes, sometimes acting together but also affected by environmental factors. Heart disease, diabetes and most cancers are examples of such disorders. Behavioral-based conditions like obesity or alcoholism, those addiction-related genes that Brody referred to in his examples, are also multifactorial.

Complicating matters, while many cancers are hereditary, cancer can also be strictly "genetic," caused by genetic mutations—that is, changes in genes that make them not work properly—not necessarily shared by family members. Scientists are now beginning to learn more about the forces behind these genetic disconnections and about how and why certain conditions affect us or pass us by. Heritage is sometimes the answer, but less so than was once believed. And people change in many ways that can't easily be accounted for. Diseases can be caused by genes, environment, behavior or chance, or by various combinations. "Humans," says Lawrence Brody, referring back to Mendel's work, "do not behave the way peas do."

There is also what is known as epigenetics (*epi* is Greek for "on or around"), which refers to factors that affect gene behavior but are actually independent of DNA sequence. That is, your genome can change as a consequence of your environment and lifestyle. In recent studies of both rats and nonhuman primates, for example, researchers have shown that affectionate mothering alters the expression of genes that help rats to handle stress more easily—a trait that is transferred to the next generation and allows that generation to more carefully nurture their offspring. The system is thought to work similarly in humans. Epigenetic factors may also hinder normal development: the offspring of parents who have withstood famine, for example, are at heightened risk for developing schizophrenia. Similar factors can mute the gene that makes the receptor for the hormone oxytocin, a substance critical in cementing relationships. There are untold complications and combinations. Examine 1,000 lung cancer patients, and you would find many recognizable and nearly identical patterns among them. But each patient's cancer would also be unique.

And yet, it is true that people generally fall into broad genetic groups that correspond with race, ethnicity and geography, and the more isolated those groups are, the more pronounced their genetic variations tend to be. The technical term is "haplotype," meaning a grouping of genetic variations, sections on strands of DNA, that tend to be passed down from generation to generation within certain populations.

The Amish, for example, who rarely marry outside their community, suffer more frequently than the general population from rare genetic diseases like dwarfism. And sickle cell anemia affects mostly those of African ancestry. Sickle cell anemia is exactly what its name says it is: people with this genetic mutation, which requires two copies of the sickle cell gene, one from each parent, have sickle-shaped (rather than normal disc-shaped) blood cells. Because of their shape, these cells don't move smoothly through blood vessels, which can result in blockages in blood flow to limbs and organs that can cause damage, strokes and, often, early death. But the sickle cell gene has a potential benefit, as well: people with only one copy of the mutation are protected against malaria, which likely explains why the mutation is common among groups who live in traditionally malarial areas.

Because Judaism is matrilineal and, until recently, Jews forcefully resisted intermarriage, the haplotype connection is startlingly apparent in Jewish populations. There are a number of genetic disorders that affect higher numbers of people in this population than any other, including Joubert syndrome type 2, which causes developmental delay in children; Bloom's syndrome, resulting in small body size and low resistance to infection and disease; Tay-Sachs and Canavan disease, both neurological disorders; and Gaucher's disease type 1, which causes a build-up of fatty tissue and weakens most organs in the body. As a result, there's a Jewish Genetic Disease Consortium that trains rabbis about how to inform and counsel their congregations, and to urge couples to undergo genetic screening before marriage.

There is also a particularly high incidence of breast cancer among Jews, and since the 1990s, much attention has been focused on the "Jewish breast cancer genes." These genes, *BRCA1* and *BRCA2* (abbreviations for breast cancer susceptibility genes 1 and 2 respectively), are defective in about 2.3% of Jewish women of Ashkenazi descent, a rate about five times higher than in the general population. A similar disparity exists with regard to ovarian cancer.

Breast cancer is an area where personalized medicine has begun to be practiced with some success. At one point in time, doctors treated all breast cancer patients with chemotherapy, an onslaught of substances toxic to growing and mutating cells and less toxic to normal cells but nevertheless often terribly destructive to the body as a whole—a situation in which the cure can be as harmful as the disease.

But breast cancer can have different causes—in some patients, the cause is an inherited genetic mutation in one of the *BRCA* genes. *BRCA1* and *BRCA2* mutations cause the majority of cases of hereditary breast cancer. *BRCA1* and *BRCA2* are tumor suppressor genes, meaning that these genes will initially protect a cell from becoming cancerous. But if the gene is mutated, cancer becomes more likely.

Breast cancer can also result from an acquired (not inherited) mutation in the HER2 (Human Epidermal growth factor Receptor 2), which is part of a pathway that signals cells to divide. It's like a relay system. The HER2 receptor gets a signal from outside the cell that says "grow," which it passes along to other proteins in the cell. The message continues to get passed on within the cell until the "grow" message gets to the nucleus (control center), and the cell begins to grow and divide. If the signal isn't stopped, that cell can keep growing and dividing; and those behaviors are part of what makes something cancer. The California-based biotech giant Genentech has developed and introduced a drug, Herceptin, which zeros in and attaches to the HER2 receptor on the outside of the cell and tells the body's immune system to knock it out. If chemo is a bombardment of the body, then Herceptin, in contrast, can be compared to a guided missile. There's a caveat, though: only about 25% of all breast cancer patients have tumors that are caused by HER2. Still, such drugs developed under the personalized medicine banner can be valuable and lifesaving.

Oncotype DX, another good example of personalized medicine, is a diagnostic test that can tell whether chemotherapy will be effective on a particular breast cancer tumor and at the same time indicate how likely it is that cancer, once in remission, may return in the future. Even though there remain many problems that need to be solved before personalized medicine becomes reality or, for that matter, before all breast cancer is eradicated or successfully treated, the success of Herceptin and Oncotype DX reflect the potential and the promise of personalized medicine—and the success of such tools has become one of the motivating factors driving the research and the expectations forward. And yet, they also reflect personalized medicine's limitations.

Trying to understand the result of a genetic test, for example, is daunting even for the geneticist. Bruce Korf at the University of Alabama compares genetic analysis to "being handed *War and Peace* and asked to find the typographical errors in the book. You start thumbing through it and maybe you will get lucky and you will see a blank page. A whole page is missing in a critical moment in the story—just like if there was a page missing in a person's genetic sequence. So that's easy. But it could be something like a misspelled word buried somewhere—and it might not even be a misspelling that creates a nonsense word. It could be a word-usage mistake, which Spell-Check would not detect, which could possibly alter the meaning of the story—the diagnosis or the translation—and the way in which you monitor and manage the disease."

To make matters even more complicated, sequencing is expensive. In 2012, whole genome sequencing costs about $10,000, and if you include handling and storage of the data that is collected and the process of interpreting it, the cost would be at least ten times higher. It's possible to look at this two ways, however: On the one hand, the price of genome sequencing has dropped dramatically—in 2007, it cost approximately $1 million. And "the $1,000 genome", which most experts consider "affordable" for patient use, will surely be achieved within the next few years. This is good. We can all be sequenced—at least those who want it and can afford it.

But on the other hand, the genome—even if sequencing it cost only $100, or $10—is not the panacea people believe it to be. For while the sequencing delivers the raw data, we have no real idea how to interpret the data or, in most cases, how to use it. Jasper Rine, a geneticist at the University of California at Berkeley, had his genome sequenced through one of the commercial genetic testing companies, which provides only a fraction of the data that would result from a whole genome sequence. "I devoted twenty hours to the printout I received," Rine told me, "to try to figure out what it all means." Then he took it to his doctor, who was able to focus fifteen minutes of his attention on it. The experience was not productive or satisfying. Genome sequencing may soon be a widely available commodity, but it may not be the silver bullet we are seeking.

And even with the information that can be gleaned from the sequence, the reality is that cancer cells are smarter than our smartest scientists—and amazingly elusive. Cancer cells have an ability referred to as "treatment resistance": that is, when they find themselves blocked in a tumor, they invariably develop another means of growth—forging a new pathway when the old pathway is blocked. Even when cancer-related mutations are discovered, it is difficult to know without intensive testing which mutations drive cancer and which happen while cancer progresses and which just happen to be present, with no connection to cancer at all. And some mutations will not respond to drugs—at least any drugs that are currently available. Targeted therapy often leads to short-lived responses. Moving these into meaningful extensions for healthy survival is a challenge as awesome as developing the therapy in the first place.

Speaking at a panel discussion, Cancer's Last Stand, the Genome Solution?, at the 2011 World Science Festival in Manhattan, Dr. Eric Lander, a Founding Director of the Broad Institute of MIT and a member of the HGP, observed, very nonscientifically, that those people who thought that cancer could be cured without a thorough understanding of the genome were, quite simply, "nuts." He added: "Let the cancer tell you what is important."

But then he added a caveat. While genetic findings have led to some very successful treatments, as with Herceptin and Gleevec, which is used successfully for targeting chronic myeloid leukemia and gastrointestinal tumors, it is misleading to assume that even successful "targeting" means "curing." This faith or reliance in the initial successes in targeting can lead to a depressing letdown. As an example, Lander referred to a drug he did not name that could magically make melanoma tumors—a deadly type of skin cancer—melt away, and disappear for nearly a year. And then, he said, the tumors come "roaring back" because the cancer develops a new mutation and simultaneously becomes resistant to the drug. So the data is nearly impossible to collect on a large-volume basis and the interpretation of the data and the subsequent therapy that may be devised can often promise more than it will in the end deliver.

A few months after the World Science Festival, a speaker at the European Multidisciplinary Cancer Congress in September 2011 summarized the challenge of understanding the genomic data that is collected after sequencing by quipping: "Genomic tests are 70% true positive, and 70% are true negative." Statisticians who will often use such terminology will tell you that both classifications are correct.

Not long after the genome was sequenced, the National Institutes of Health began funding genome-wide association studies—GWAS or "Geewahs." The idea behind GWAS is to get back to basics and use evidence-based medicine to examine and prove connections between genes and disease—and to ascertain the worth of the investment in future research and development of diagnostic and treatment drugs. Just like other epidemiological studies, GWAS examine large populations of people in the United States and abroad with a certain disease, comparing their DNA with that of people—subjects—who don't have the disease.

We have known for a long time that there are genetic links to rare or "orphan" diseases which do not attract very much public attention, in part because they affect fewer than 200,000 people, worldwide. But GWAS were designed to deal with the more common diseases—like heart failure, cancer, late-onset diabetes and Alzheimer's—that affect millions of people worldwide

Thousands of GWAS have been conducted over the past five years, and are continuing to be conducted, and mountains of data collected and analyzed. By 2010, more than 1,500 disease-related genes had been discovered, and 1,300 genetic tests developed for conditions ranging from hearing loss to sudden cardiac death. In addition to advances in breast cancer diagnosis and treatment, the sequencing of the genome has led to the discovery of a genetic variant leading to age-related macular degeneration, a major cause of blindness. Genetic linkages have been discovered for type 2 diabetes, Parkinson's disease and Crohn's disease, and GWAS may eventually lead to the development of drugs that can fight or prevent lupus. But this is just a drop in the bucket—and, unfortunately, none of the connections are definitive. Genetic variants have been linked to disease—but they only add up to a modest connection between DNA and risk for the disease. The connection is surprisingly small, perhaps only one tenth of the total heritability of a disease. As an example, scientists believe that the heritability of height is as much as 80% genetic, but until recently, science could prove genetic heritability of only 5%. In 2010, however, a team led by scientists at the Queensland Institute of Medical Research in Australia found that when a large number of genetic variations were considered together, the proof level increased to 45%. With data amassed by the predicted inexpensive genetic sequencing tools which may be available by 2015, they suspect that proof level may increase to 50%.

In addition, more than one gene may be connected to a disease. For example, 20 variants have so far been discovered for type 2 diabetes, explaining only 6% of the disease. Genetic linkages to Crohn's can be traced to only 15% of the victims. Not significant. Some experts counter the pessimism displayed by these low numbers, by maintaining that 6% and 15% are beginnings, breakthroughs, and even small percentages signify hope.

But GWAS have not provided a great deal of clarity, unless you want to say that knowledge came from what physicists call "dark matter"—meaning that because we could not draw definitive conclusions, we have learned enough to know that we have a lot more to learn

So, GWAS have been helpful if not conclusive, according to some experts who feel that as the research continues more common variants will be found and, in time, we will be able to target those variants and make an impact on a given disease. Other experts counter this argument by maintaining that as we continue to research we will discover more risk-causing variants, making it virtually impossible to find the path between cause and effect—between gene and disease. One geneticist, David B. Goldstein at Duke University, uses schizophrenia as an example: There may be 1,000 rather than 100 or even 10 rare genetic variants that cause the disease—meaning that the genetic route to schizophrenia would be, in a sense, schizophrenic. Build in epigenetics and other unpredictable factors, and untangling the complications in any schizophrenia scenario would be unimaginable.

Still, although most scientists agree that the HGP was far from a waste— scientists learned a lot about our basic biology—the knowledge has not to any degree filtered down to the point where doctors could do a lot with it for their patients—or at least so doctors thought. Many critics were asking (and continue to ask): "So what's the genome done for us lately?"

This is not such a fair question, and it is shortsighted, at best. Consider the larger picture. Before the beginning of the twentieth century human lifespan increased by only twenty years over a 4,000-year period. In the twentieth century alone, lifespan was increased by thirty years—and it was a process. At the turn of the century, we found aspirin; in the 1940s, we began to use penicillin; in the 1960s researchers discovered that chemotherapy can effectively kill cancer cells; and in the 1980s, the era of transplantation began, progressing from kidney to bone marrow to face transplants. Now, we are moving into the era of personalized medicine, but it will be gradual, like most major transformations. Computers have been in popular use since the 1970s, for example, but only today are we beginning to realize the amazing impact—from Facebook to smart phones—the computer has had and will continue to have on society. The personalized medicine transition, many geneticists point out, will contain not just one "P" word—but four: not just personalized, but predictive, preventive and participatory medicine.

It is that last "P"—for "participatory"—that may well be most crucial and that will move personalized medicine forward so that the research can become connected with real-life patients.

CHAPTER 3:
FAMILY HISTORIES

In 1948, the National Heart, Lung and Blood Institute (NHLBI), then called the National Heart Institute, launched a study of more than 5,000 men and women aged thirty to sixty-two, all from the town of Framingham, Massachusetts, who had not yet developed overt symptoms of cardiovascular disease or suffered a heart attack or stroke. Three successive generations have been involved in follow-up studies, the idea being that careful monitoring would lead to the identification of major cardiovascular disease risk factors, as well as information on the effects of factors such as blood pressure, blood triglyceride and cholesterol levels, age, gender and psychosocial issues, among other things. What is today considered common knowledge in relation to heart disease was isolated and confirmed in this manner. However, the Framingham Risk Score, which is based on this research and has been used for many years to estimate a person's chances of having a heart attack, did not take family history into account. As a result, the score was of limited use for patients who fell into a gray area, by exhibiting some, but not all, of the Framingham risk factors.

In 2007, a new risk model, the Reynolds Risk Score, was introduced, which includes family history in the calculation. The Reynolds study initially focused on women, collecting information from 24,000 females over the course of a decade and comparing their Framingham Risk Score with their actual medical history—that is, whether they actually had a heart attack. The inclusion of family history information resulted in the reclassification of nearly 50% of those women as at risk for cardiac problems. In a second, smaller study of more than 1,700 men, 20% of the male subjects were also reclassified. By not including family history as a risk factor, the Framingham study was missing half of the people at risk.

Someday family histories will be routine, as they should be today—the first event of a patient's interaction with a physician. A complete family history should take at least forty-five minutes and go back as far in time as a patient's memory allows. Under the best of conditions, family members should be consulted before and after the history is taken to expand the details and help the medical staff make less obvious connections.

But why go through the trouble of getting a family history? Why not just invest a few hundred dollars in one of those online genomic testing services that analyze DNA glitches and predict people's predisposition to various diseases? A recent study at the Cleveland Clinic provided an answer by recruiting twenty-two cancer patients and their spouses—forty-four people in all—and taking each subject's family history, as well as doing the genetic testing. The spouses served as the control group. Both the genetic tests and the family histories indicated that 40% of the cancer patients were at above-average risk for colon cancer—but they didn't identify the same people. The genetic screening missed all nine people whose histories indicated a strong risk.

The thing about family histories is that few patients volunteer for them. In part, this is because most patients don't really know what a family history actually is; you might assume, for instance, when a nurse's aide enters the exam room and asks questions about your health, that he or she is taking a history—and, to a certain extent, that's true. Many doctors may assume this is the extent of a family history, as well. And even if a doctor does know what a complete family history is, it is difficult to find a doctor willing to commit the time needed for a thorough interview, and follow-up interviews with family members, and making sense of the results; the economics of the healthcare system don't encourage such undertakings.

As a practical matter, most family histories are given in response to serious illness, often after it's too late to help the patient. By that time, the patient may feel he or she has more important problems, like staying alive and getting well, and so the physician and the coordinator often have a difficult time persuading patients to follow up and do the kind of testing that might help shed light on a family legacy and bring information and guidance to other family members.

Once taken, the family history should be constantly updated with new information about parents, spouses, cousins and other family members as standard operating procedure throughout the doctor's relationship with the patient. But today, most family histories tend to be done in a large medical center, usually precipitated by a serious illness. Usually, genetic counselors see patients who may be interested in family histories and genetic testing. There are few, if any, genetic counselors employed by general practitioners or family-practice physicians—at least not yet.

Different than nurses or physicians' assistants, genetic counselors have completed a master's-level program in medical genetics and in counseling skills. They must pass a certification exam administered by the American Board of Genetic Counseling in order to practice. They, rather than physicians, conduct most family histories and help families identify and interpret risks of inherited disorders. They explain inheritance patterns, and suggest possible testing for mutations and outline possible scenarios so that families can more thoroughly understand the process and the science of genetics. Also trained in counseling, they can address emotional issues raised by the results of the genetic testing.

Over the past few years, I have observed a number of family histories. They all seem to follow the same general rhythm, with the doctor or the genetic counselor gently probing the patient or family members for information concerning their family background and roots: where the family comes from, the health of cousins and uncles, siblings and parents. It is a search for sickness and wellness.

Uncle Joe? He had emphysema. Worked in the mines.

Cousin Sophie? She died at fifteen of a brain tumor—a gorgeous girl.

My daddy lived until ninety—smoked two packs a day, but never sick a day in his life.

My mother was tired and took a nap. Never woke up.

Uncle Albert went on a run, came home, walked into the living room, yelled up the stairs to my aunt, "Honey, I'm back!" and immediately dropped dead.

The genetic coordinator or doctor taking a family history practices in a manner similar to a psychotherapist—keeping the conversation going, focusing on the patient, asking pertinent questions, nodding and encouraging the patient and other family members, if they're present, to contribute—all the while drawing stick figures on an artist's sketch pad of each actor mentioned (mother, brother, etc.) and connecting the stick figures with colored arrows that represent relationships and diseases.

The history eventually resembles a complicated patchwork quilt of familial connections—how complicated depends on the depth of the patient's memories, the size of the family and the skill and persistence of the interrogator. Most genetic counselors use a computer program to turn their stick-figure scribblings into a graphic, full-color chart, which they print out and mail to the patient not long after the family history takes place—a memorable gesture, and a valuable document.

Almost always, a family history is the precursor to genetic testing. In some ways, there's a conflict of interest here: one way or another, the medical center, the physician and the coordinator benefit when patients agree to undergo testing.

There's the obvious income that goes to the lab if the test is hospital-based, and invariably the tests are also part of research studies being conducted by the medical staff. I am not saying that patients are being misled, necessarily—but there's a push and pull here to be noted.

Michael Saks, the law professor, was not particularly excited about reaching out to his relatives to gather information—his was not a close-knit family—but his desire to discover as much as possible about his vulnerability to pancreatic cancer convinced him to cooperate. He made friendly catching-up phone calls to his relatives, ostensibly checking in with family members to see how everyone was feeling and what they were doing, so that he would be able to answer the questions he expected Hunt would ask. As a researcher himself, he knew he would have to buy into the process if it was to work. But he never told his relatives that he was preparing to undergo a family history and blood work for medical reasons—perhaps because it did not seem worth the trouble and perhaps, also, because it might seem self-serving to his cousins.

Later, he would be taken to task for involving his family in his own genetic testing—or at least the way in which he went about doing it.

I was unable to observe Michael Saks's family history with Katherine Hunt, but I have observed many other family histories, conducted by different physicians and genetic counselors. Here are parts of two such family histories:

Room #1

"You were diagnosed about six years ago?" the counselor asks the man sitting across from her.

"Yes." Dennis, her patient, in his early forties, has been diagnosed with retinized pigmentosa, a group of genetically related eye conditions that cause irreversible blindness.

"At that time, what sort of issues were you having?"

"What do you mean?" Dennis asks.

"Do you have trouble with night blindness, for example?"

"I am not driving anymore because at night the lights from the oncoming cars hit me in the face and I can't see. I have also lost some peripheral vision. I bump my head on cabinets regularly."

"Do you see shadings between colors?"

"Colors of the rainbow, reds and oranges run together on the right eye—black and white only on the left eye."

Dennis is balding, with frameless glasses. He has been sick for a long time with kidney disease, he says. The complications are frustrating. "Makes you weary," he says.

"How did you first realize you were having sight problems?"

"I was taking a math class," he says. "I took a test. I am pretty good at math—it comes easy—but for this test I was crossing my equal signs and minus signs, so that they looked like pluses or number signs. So the teacher came and said, 'You failed, and that is not like you. You are too smart to fail.' So I thought about it for a while and eventually got an eye examination. That is when I realized what was happening—probably because of my kidneys."

"You've had trouble with kidneys?"

"My kidney was starting to shrivel up—a long time ago. I was on dialysis for a year, until I got an eleven-month-old pediatric kidney in a transplant. Actually, they put two pediatric kidneys in me at one time and I did well for six years."

"And then what happened?"

"I picked up Epstein-Barr virus, and we went back and forth trying to keep the kidneys, me and my doctors. We are still going back and forth, still struggling."

While she is questioning Dennis, the counselor is making a chart of health issues and family members, essentially Dennis's medical family tree. She will eventually turn the chart into a full-color computerized printout, which she will send to him.

Dennis has come prepared. He has interviewed his mother and his wife and has some interesting information to communicate, he says. He and his wife share the same last name, but he has done some independent genealogical research in the old country, Ireland, and is fairly certain that there is no direct family connection.

At the end of the interview, Dennis has two decisions to make related to testing. He could walk away and choose not to find out more about his condition. Or he could choose between a clinical test, for which his insurance company will pay, or research testing. Results from clinical testing will come within the next few weeks. Data from the research study will also be shared—but much later. "A long time," says the counselor.

Testing for retinized pigmentosa does not always identify causative mutations. No matter what he chooses, Dennis may not receive the answers he is seeking.

Dennis chooses the fast track. "Too much going on in my life that I don't understand," he says. "The more I know—information I can get—the more secure I will be."

Room #2

Jessica is wearing a purple baseball cap with yellow, red and pink polka dots, a black knee-length coat, blue jeans and running shoes. She is bald, like most cancer patients receiving chemotherapy. She says, with a twangy southern lilt, that she is fifty-seven years old—"and getting older by the treatment." Jessica is hesitant to advise her daughter, Jill, a thirty-eight-year-old single mom, to take the BRCA test. They have come together to the oncology clinic to talk about Jill's options with a doctor and genetic counselor. Jessica thought that the doctor should advise her daughter.

Jill, sitting beside her mother in a straight-backed wooden chair, has two daughters of her own. She works in a nearby medical center, so she is perhaps more informed than the average family member or patient. But the knowledge makes her leery and elicits questions that seem to reflect ambivalence and uncertainty.

"Are the results of this test going to be part of my official medical history?" Jill asks. "I am worried that everyone will know about me. It will be in my chart—my record. I mean," she says, "will there be discrimination against me? People won't want to hire me because I could get breast cancer and need medical coverage and maybe not be able to work."

"There's legislation," says the counselor. "The Genetic Nondiscrimination Act. GINA. Not to worry," she adds.

"But they could force me to take a genetic test," says Jill.

"Who would force you to take a test?"

"My employer or my insurance carrier." She laughs, "I don't know—God knows who!"

"No, they can't. Insurance companies or employers can't require genetic testing or use any of the information to turn you down for coverage or increase what you pay for coverage. They can't even give lower rates to

employees who voluntarily give their family histories to prove how healthy they are—and will be."

"Does GINA go into effect for life insurance?"

"No, it does not, I am sorry to say."

"My mother has this breast cancer mutation," says Jill, "and you say that there's a 50-50 chance that I will have it. But what if I don't have it? Does that mean that my daughters won't have it? Are they off the hook?"

"Not necessarily."

"I don't know," says Jill, "there's a lot to find out."

"Your mother has had breast cancer," says the doctor, who has been listening quietly, "and has taken the initiative and had a double mastectomy, which is a good thing. I mean—" he says, suddenly realizing that his sentence didn't necessarily come out the way in which he had intended, "I certainly don't want to imply that having this mutation is a good thing. This is something I would not sign up for. But knowing about it is a good thing. We are now armed with information because you"—he turns to Jessica—"took the initiative, as I said. By having a mastectomy you have effectively decreased your risk for future breast cancer, to a dramatic extent."

Jessica nods and smiles sympathetically, understanding that what he is saying is true, but the conversation is awkward. Or perhaps the way in which he speaks is awkward. He is a physician and an academic, and very often his words come out sounding kind of stilted.

"The good thing about finding this mutation is that now we know what is going on. There is no more mystery. What remains is how we deal with that increased risk of ovarian cancer. While we doctors are decent at detecting breast cancer, we are not good at detecting ovarian cancer, and therefore I am being directive in telling you what should be done, and I am being very straightforward. I think you should have your ovaries removed. You have a lot of years ahead of you—you are only fifty-seven years old. You have a lot of life to live." He pauses.

He has been focusing all of his attention on the mother, but now he turns to Jill, the daughter. "Let's talk about you for a minute. There are, in fact, women who say, 'No way, I am not going to have a mastectomy,' and I say, 'Fine, okay, we've got plan B and we will go from there.' And then there are other women who tell me, 'I already have an appointment with a surgeon.'

"Of course, I understand that none of these decisions might have to be made by you now because in fact you have a 50% chance of not having a

mutation, which means that you have a 50% chance of being cancer free. So this is all to the good.

"But when it comes to your ovaries, I would be as adamant with you as I have been with your mom. From the breast cancer standpoint, there are decent options: Bilateral mastectomy and reconstructive surgery. Another reasonable choice is surveillance—with lumpectomy—although not as effective." He pauses and then adds: "I think you should get tested now—let us take blood now. Then we can go from there."

"I wonder," says Jill, "if there are false positives to this test?"

"A great question—but no. I feel very confident that the result we got from your mother is not a false positive. She has the mutation."

"Is there anyone," asked Jill, "doing anything about fixing the gene?"

"Well, yes, work and research are going on all the time, but it is an unbelievably challenging engineering problem. Your body consists of three billion cells, and just in your breast there are millions of cells. You would have to fix this in every one of those cells. It is science fiction at this point."

"Will it ever be done?"

"I think it is possible—someday—but not in time for my kids or your kids."

"What happens if I have my breasts removed and my ovaries removed? Is there still a chance that it will come back in other parts of my body?"

"Another good question. It is not the situation that by taking the breasts off and removing the ovaries you squeeze this mutation into other organs. Doesn't work like that."

"Okay. I see."

"Look, you will have dramatically reduced the risk of cancer by doing those two things—tests to see if you have the breast cancer mutation and removing your ovaries. Does it eliminate the possibility of you getting cancer? No. But I would say that by doing those two things you are at a lower risk than the general population."

"I have a daughter eleven years old," says Jill.

"When she is eighteen, twenty years old, then we want to sit down and talk with her—the landscape may have changed by then in relation to testing, but she too has a chance of having the mutation, so when she gets older she ought to talk with us."

"Well, let me think about all you have told me," Jill says.

"Take your time," the doctor replies.

CHAPTER 4:
THE SHERPA

At a personalized medicine conference I attended in 2010, about 200 social workers, physicians, hospital administrators, nurses and others listened for two days to presentations concerning the potential of personalized medicine in a variety of applications—from kidney disease to diabetes. But near the end of the second day, at the final Q and A—after the last of the presentations, in fact—an elderly man with gray hair and a body too small for his suit walked up to the microphone.

"I've practiced medicine for many, many years," he said, "and I know that personalized medicine can be very, very good." He paused and looked up at the speakers. "But that's not real world. The real world is people who can't see doctors for two or three months at a time. The real world is filled with patients who need to see cardiologists—and can't. The real world for me," he said, "is that there is no time to spend with patients."

As is often the case when doctors in the trenches criticize researchers who are not mostly clinicians, there followed a deafening silence.

Steve Murphy, "The Gene Sherpa," was not at that conference. But he should have been. He would have stood up and bravely attacked not only this private-practice physician, no matter how sincere, for his reluctance to think out of the box, but also the scientists in attendance, for being equally off base, self-absorbed and suffering from research tunnel vision—thinking only of the science and not the people who may someday be helped by the science.

Murphy believed that personalized medicine was the way of the future for the healthcare world and he, then only a few years past his residency, was the missing link between the two groups—not the first physician to intimately understand genetics, but the first, significantly, to establish a personalized medicine private practice. At that moment, he wasn't quite certain how to reach the researchers, isolated from the real world in their "ivy-covered towers," but he knew that he could help the general practice physician see more patients and care for them more efficiently and personally, using a personalized medicine approach. In 2010, Murphy's newly established practice was in the doldrums, on the edge of failure, but nevertheless he had unwavering self-confidence and faith in his approach, coupled with a willingness to seek help in the social media arena.

Day Zero . . . from **The Sherpa**

> OK, so I have no idea where to begin. Which is why I will just start with the stats . . . Only 17% of patients with familial colon cancer risk were referred to appropriate genetic counseling according to <u>a study at Harvard.</u>
> Prenatal counseling is not offered to nine of ten women who meet indications!
> **Only 37% of MDs** know that BRCA genes can be passed by the father!
> We have a lot to cover and I look forward to sharing my solution to this huge problem.
> How in the world can we expect to implement Personalized Medicine in all its glory without having some Genome Savvy physicians? Oh. . ..Those geneticists? Too bad almost 90% are pediatricians and have no clue what ischemic heart failure is.

I first met Steve Murphy while doing my initial personalized medicine research online. Not much had been written about the subject in magazines or books, but there were a surprising number of bloggers weighing in, most of whom were young people: graduate students and a few post-docs, all of them fascinated by and quite optimistic about what genetics and personalized medicine could bring to the world in the coming decade. Murphy was optimistic, too—more so than most, in fact—but he was also angry at everyone: geneticists, pharmaceutical companies, DNA testing companies, you name it . . . In his blog, he let them all have it, setting the tone in his first few posts, using a few salient statistics to get some attention and to make a point. Most of his first posts were a steady salvo of attacks against detractors and nonbelievers, including doctors, counselors and teachers and all the colleagues who had spurned him or, worse, ignored genetics and personalized medicine. Murphy was blunt, maybe even a little desperate in tone. You could tell that he was trying to attract attention, but he also had a message that seemed to resonate with people from many walks of life:

> Internists don't know what the hell they're doing, genetic counselors don't know what they're doing—they think they know a lot about medicine and step over their bounds—academic people won't teach genetics 'cause they don't know anything about it or they are too busy to try to learn.

He went on and on in his posts, just as (I soon discovered) he does in real life, when you sit and talk with him over coffee. Murphy won't actually drink the coffee—and he won't actually eat, if you go out to lunch with him—because he is so obsessed with genetics and personalized medicine; he would rather pontificate and lash out, or climb up on a soapbox, than drink or eat. When it comes to genetics and personalized medicine, he's a squawking, can't-stop-talking machine.

But that approach works well online, and Murphy's blog was attracting many followers—like me. He quickly received a lot of feedback from his Sherpa persona. People remembered The Gene Sherpa and recognized Murphy's name at conferences, and his reputation was fortified by his connection to Yale, where he was working on a genetics fellowship, especially since he also pulled no punches about the lack of real knowledge and interest in genetics at Yale. To put it mildly, he was not making a lot of friends, but he was causing a bit of commotion, which was all to the good, as he saw it.

Not that his was the only genetics and personalized medicine blog; as I said, many counselors, PhD researchers and informed and concerned citizens were speaking out. But Murphy was a doctor. This was special. His MD provided rare credibility in the personalized medicine blogosphere at that time. Plus, he was so obviously passionate, as well as angry, in a field where passion in public is rare. And he was no slick media type; unlike Dr. Phil or Dr. Oz, he sounded like a real person.

Murphy is not a very good writer; he can't or won't go to the trouble to spell or punctuate correctly, and, as the Sherpa, at least, he is sometimes somewhat juvenile and maybe even a little scatological. He sometimes uses acronyms; thus, some of the points he attempts to make don't make a lot of sense to the uninformed. But the basic bluntness that accompanied his Sherpa posts, along with his off-the-cuff remarks, was remarkably genuine and appealing. Like Howard Beale from the movie *Network*, Murphy's persona was *mad as hell* that personalized medicine and genetics were not endorsed and adopted by the world at large, and he didn't hesitate to shout his complaints and objections from the rooftops. *And I'm not gonna take this anymore.* Murphy is referred to by some of his detractors (and fans) as "The Howard Stern of Genomics."

But, you might ask, who or what is the Gene Sherpa? I mean, really? His website tells you:

> To usher in the new paradigm of personalized medicine we will need to travel a perilous path. Much like the route through the Himalayas it has punished the naive and self-reliant. That is why I have dedicated my life to being a Gene Sherpa. What is a gene sherpa? The Sherpa speaks the language of the trail, he/she knows shortcuts and dangerous paths to avoid. This blog is for those wishing to take the journey and those wishing to become gene sherpas.

I had no wish to be a sherpa, actually. But I did reach out to Murphy, and we scheduled a meeting in the spring of 2007, more than a half-dozen years after the pomp, circumstance and celebration of the White House event. We rendezvoused at Murphy's swanky Park Avenue office, a small space he had leased from another doctor in Manhattan to use for two afternoons a week, for $2,000 per month. But after we shook hands, he immediately led me out the door, explaining that he had to see a referral patient to conduct a family history—not a particularly challenging task for a young MD, but after all, he said, he was building a new practice.

Murphy is handsome and youthful—he was thirty-one at that time—with thick, rumpled, black hair and an easy smile that brightens his baby-blue eyes and invariably brings flushes of color to his cheeks. In Greenwich Hospital, where he sees patients and has served two residencies, he often wears baggy polo shorts or sweaters and loose-fitting trousers that make him seem more like a medical student than a full-fledged professional. He's clearly more himself in casual attire, comfortable and spontaneous, but that day he was wearing a white shirt, a green-and-black-striped tie and brown shoes. He's always slightly disheveled. His shirt is never quite tucked in and his scuffed shoes have probably never been polished.

He's a fast walker, necessarily in a hurry, racing from one place to another, sidestepping pedestrians and texting as he walks. We took off toward the patient's primary care doctor's office, Murphy talking rapid-fire between texts about how no one in internal medicine pays any attention to genetics and how sorry they will be when they realize the medical world has left them far behind and how difficult it will be for them to catch up, when I ran into an old friend—a journalist who, knowing that I live out of town, immediately asked: "What are you doing here?"

"I am working on a story about personalized medicine," I told him and, nodding in Murphy's direction, explained, "I am interviewing Dr. Steve Murphy. He's a personalized medicine doctor—maybe the first in private practice—ever."

My friend scrunched his eyes quizzically and responded. "My doctor is very personal with me. I can call him up any time—or go and see him—and we talk."

Murphy was running late. But later, he referred back to our encounter with my friend to illustrate the trouble he was having getting his personalized medicine practice off the ground: "Not a lot of people realize what personalized medicine is all about. Not just patients. You ask some doctors what personalized medicine means—and they give defensive or evasive answers, like: 'Are you saying I don't pay attention to my patients? That I am not personal enough?' Or they fish for clues: 'Personalized medicine? That has something to do with genetics, doesn't it?'"

This encounter with my friend on Park Avenue and Steve Murphy's frustration represent one of the inherent problems of this new era of medicine called "personalized medicine." In many ways, it begins with the term itself, which is so vague it can be molded to fit into anyone's general conception—and also inherently suggests something negative about many doctors.

The term, says Bruce Korf, implies the existence of "impersonalized medicine": "A lot of doctors would say, 'What have I been practicing all these years? I see patients one at a time, and I try to deal with their personal issues when I see them, so isn't that personalized medicine?'" Korf is not being disingenuous, but perhaps he is being overly generous. Surveys indicate that the average contact time between patient and physician is anywhere from seven to twelve minutes. True, medical schools teach that listening to a patient's story is a primary key to diagnosis—but that's not a lot of time for conversation.

The imprecision of the term and the way in which it can be molded to suit almost any circumstance became quite clear to me as I interviewed physicians, researchers, hospital and medical school administrators, residents and others. Before I began asking questions, my subject would invariably want to clarify: "Let me ask you first, what do *you* mean by personalized medicine?" These nurses and doctors were seeking some direction—*What is it that this reporter really wants to talk about?* When pressed, I would usually reply with an umbrella definition, beginning with genomics and ending with pharmacology, hitting as many bases as possible in between, which is easy with such a generic label— until I touched a chord of recognition. Clearly, personalized medicine could mean anything the interviewee was most interested in—and the definitions and examples I heard in interviews were wide ranging.

When asked for her definition of personalized medicine, a nurse who admits patients at a high-acuity cancer center explained that when patients call she asks for their name, punches it into the computer and then chats them up about the personal matters she has heard and collected and has stored in the computer, making them feel comfortable, "part of the family." That's personalized medicine. The associate dean of a medical school that promotes personalized medicine downplays genetics but stresses "biomedical informatics"—basically, using computers to share information, worldwide, about patients, research and medications to enhance the individualization and effectiveness of treatment.

Dr. Ken Buetow, director of the National Cancer Institute Center for Bioinformatics and Information Technology, sees personalized medicine as "the right information at the right time." Buetow appeared at a forum about personalized medicine in Washington, at which the results of a poll of 800 adults were announced, showing that only 5% of the recipients connected the term *personalized medicine* with DNA. Buetow was asked how he might have responded, had he been polled. "I probably would have hemmed and hawed a little bit," he replied, "because I think . . . there's not a crisp, singular definition. But the one that best grasps for me, I guess, would be the integrated use of diverse information to learn about an individual and their disease and to prevent and treat the disease."

A physician from a large medical center in New York asked for my definition of personalized medicine before starting our interview, then told me the title of the talk he was giving at meeting in Texas: The Advent of Genomic Medicine— Hope, Hype and Reality.

The "hype" is a major problem, according the ethicist and director of the Center for Law and the Biosciences at Stanford University, Hank Greely: personalized medicine "is a wonderful term—rolls smoothly off your tongue—it sounds good. Who could be against personalized medicine? The alternative is what? Impersonal medicine? But are we allowing personalized medicine to be overhyped or hyping it ourselves? What we see in the newspapers and magazines and out in the market is hype—and hype, almost by definition, is an ethical problem."

For the most part, people know that the sequencing of the human genome has occurred, and they have a basic understanding of what that means—although, as Craig Venter has noted, the jury is still out in relation to whether this accomplishment will be perceived with positive or negative connotations. Ethics and legalities are only now being entered into the mix of discussion and debate. But few patients—and their doctors—connect genetics with the label, *personalized medicine*, that has been adopted to describe this future way of practicing medicine.

This was only one of many stumbling blocks Murphy was to encounter in his attempt to set up a personalized medicine practice. Looking back at the recent history of the personalized medicine movement, however, no one—except maybe Francis Collins—has worked harder than Steve Murphy at promoting the personalized medicine mission and message. Murphy was kind of crazy, you might say, in the way he unrelentingly came at you, with opinions, statistics and jargon. But what else would you expect from a true believer?

CHAPTER 5:
RANTING AND RAVING
AND GOING NOWHERE

Ok, so today is one of those little rant days. I am pretty sick and tired of companies, politicians and bankers . . . It just plain stinks that our economy hit the skids. But we did a lot of this to ourselves. How? Some **say Greed**. Others say **lack of regulations**.

I say, **we believed in Bull$h!t** . . . **Everyone was selling it** . . . That is what killed this economy.

Think about it, our intuitive **BS meters were dropped a long time ago**. Million dollar homes in rural America???? Sure, why not? Everywhere else prices are going up . . . Only make 50k a year? That's ok, your house is worth that million . . . We'll take that risk.

The same thing was true with Biotech and this new abomination of DTC . . . Have a technology that has no true clinical application, nor proven utility for informing people of risk???? Sounds great. Here's your term sheet . . . heck, why not? Everyone else is doing it . . .

This type of overselling killed the mortgage industry. It destroyed the market . . . And like Francis Collins had said in the past, over selling personalized medicine is the quickest way to destroy its promise . . .

But, don't worry about me folks . . . My bull$h!t meter is back on and ticking . . .

In 2007, Steve Murphy could clearly see all of the red flags warning him to go slowly and consider holding off on starting his personalized medicine practice for another few years. He repeated them to me often: His colleagues were not buying into genetics, let alone personalized medicine, and would therefore not be sending him the needed referrals; he was new in the business and really didn't know anybody to help him make connections, meet other doctors and sell himself; the privacy laws in relation to genetic information were unclear, and people were afraid to share or "go public" because of the possible consequences; even if patients wanted to share their genetic information, their health insurance might not pay for the testing, so they'd have to come up with their own hard, cold cash; the stock market was crashing, and even the super-rich folks on the Upper East Side of Manhattan, where Murphy had located his practice, or in plush, lush Greenwich, Connecticut, where he had a second office, were thinking two and three times about spending money, seeing how their personal fortunes had diminished significantly; and even in the best of times, Murphy, all alone, could not easily cover two practices, commute forty minutes each way between Greenwich and Manhattan, share childcare duties with his wife (also a physician), and commute forty minutes in a different direction to New Haven to see patients and do research at Yale, where he was in the first year of a three-year personalized medicine fellowship which he had designed for himself.

Even Murphy's mentor had serious doubts about his ability to pull all this off. According to Dr. Charles Seelig, director of resident education at Greenwich Hospital, Steve Murphy was brilliant and he had charisma, and his deep-seated knowledge of genetics was impressive. One meeting with Murphy had persuaded Seelig to change part of the curriculum of the residency program at the hospital to reflect a heavy emphasis on genetics, with Murphy leading the way. "I knew immediately that he was different than the average resident—filled with passion and drive and a hunger for change," Seelig recalls. "And he knew more as a student about genetics than most doctors know when they have finished all of their training."

Seelig requisitioned hospital funds so he and Murphy could take a seminar focusing on personalized medicine at Harvard and bring back the information to share with all the doctors in a series of lectures. For a relatively small local hospital to make such a radical change—delving into an obscure field, pioneered by a physician-resident who had never practiced outside of his residency and was not yet boarded in genetics or internal medicine—was unusual, to say the least. But Murphy was that persuasive, says Seelig: "You look for this spark of desire and commitment in young doctors, but rarely do you see it. Here was a kid devoted to an idea and willing to sacrifice his life—it was irresistible." But Seelig also thought Murphy was jumping in too fast, and he warned Murphy that he might be making a huge mistake—and losing more lucrative opportunities.

"I was offered a position with a physician in town who does concierge medicine," Murphy once told me. Concierge (or "boutique") medicine is a retainer-based system in which patients pay doctors a monthly or annual fee, usually out of pocket, to receive personalized attention and care. (In this case, "personalized" refers to special treatment and guaranteed access to the doctor; concierge practices usually limit the number of patients they accept.) "He wanted to start me at $250,000 with a potential bonus, but I wouldn't be doing what I want to do, and would not be permitted to talk about personalized medicine," Murphy explained. Even his wife wanted him to take the job, but neither spouse nor mentor could dissuade Murphy from going off on his own.

Murphy acknowledged that he was gambling with his future—but he was on a mission. Personalized medicine would be the launching point of his career and his future—and that was that, as far as Murphy was concerned. No matter what others said, he believed he was jumping in at the tipping point. Personalized medicine would soon be embraced by doctors, patients, pharmaceutical companies, state and federal government—and he would be there first. He envisioned this clearly in his mind: himself as part of a brotherhood of true believers. Francis Collins preached personalized medicine to scientists in their research towers and legislators in Washington, while he, Steve Murphy, was in the trenches of general practice, beseeching his colleagues to pay attention to the future of medicine, the *personalized* future—if not for themselves, then for their patients.

Murphy was clearly driven and genuinely obsessed, but he also seemed cavalier and inexplicably overconfident, it seemed to me. Granted, he was willing to concede that his youth and lack of contacts in Manhattan were working against him on Park Avenue; as large and diverse as New York is, there was a definite medical hierarchy that he could not easily penetrate.

But he was puzzled by the lack of interest—and business—in Greenwich. He had, after all, served two residencies at Greenwich Hospital. He had been chief resident one of those years, and very popular with the medical staff. He had persuaded Dr. Seelig to allow him to teach genetics classes to the medical staff.

"All these guys, doctors, knew me from the hospital," Murphy said, "but why weren't they referring to me?" It was so terribly frustrating. Why couldn't he reach them? How could they not see the future of medicine right in front of their eyes? Had they never heard of the Human Genome Project? Didn't they read medical journals? What about the stories in the *New York Times*? Their heads were in the sand—or in their profit-and-loss statements.

This is why he had created the Gene Sherpa persona. In fact, on one of those occasions when I visited Steve Murphy on Park Avenue, early on, I noticed that he was carrying a book with a familiar bright yellow color and design. I asked him what he was reading and, blushing more than a little sheepishly, he held it up for me to see: *PUBLIC RELATIONS FOR DUMMIES*.

"The book said I should blog—get your name on the Internet, it said. Find your voice and tell people what you want to do. Declare yourself!" Murphy told me. "The book said that in the blog you should write down things you want to do related to the message you want to convey and get started. So I did that— just as they suggested."

I nodded. I didn't know what to say.

"Well," he said finally. "It's a start."

It turned out to be a good start. The blog helped him establish a voice and a presence in the personalized medicine world, though he still had very few patients. So in an effort to improve his communication—and business— Murphy engaged a marketing team to help him understand why his practice was not catching on. Here the interviews conducted by the marketing company were eliciting important information—information which was frustrating to hear, but not necessarily surprising. Murphy's colleagues were not antagonistic to him; rather, they were clueless. When asked if they were familiar with personalized medicine, they replied predictably: 'That is when you are on twenty-four-hour call.' Or, 'That is when you see patients and talk with them.' Some version of that idea," Murphy said. "Or that it is concierge medicine.

"This was very frustrating," Murphy said. But it wasn't just the fact that Murphy's colleagues didn't recognize or understand the personalized medicine label—they also didn't get what he was doing. They knew, more or less, what geneticists did in major medical centers, and they had been made familiar with genetics during the first two years of medical school. Nature versus nurture was constantly debated, and it didn't take a medical-school education to know that both are major influences in shaping a human being. Still, Murphy's colleagues couldn't quite see how genetics might benefit their patients.

"Yes, I know Steve does genetics," the doctors in Greenwich told the marketing folks, "but I still don't know what he does. What does he do with genetics? How can I refer my patients to him in good conscience if I don't, at the very baseline, know why?"

"They couldn't wrap themselves around the idea of how a private-practice geneticist might serve their patients," Murphy speculated.

Perhaps they also couldn't wrap themselves around the idea of sharing their patients with another physician—especially when that physician was riding the wave of what some consider an oncoming, game-changing force.

Physicians, Murphy said, are aware of—and protective of—their turf. He wasn't telling me anything I hadn't noticed during my four years observing the transplant world. The tensions between the heart surgeon and the cardiologist or the liver transplant surgeon and/or kidney transplant surgeon and the gastroenterologist and urologist were ongoing and often mean—and sometimes ruinous to the losing party—and not in any way beneficial to the patient. These people played for keeps. In a follow-up book I wrote about a children's hospital, I found that the pediatricians, even though they had many different specialties, worked together much more closely. The lives of helpless children are dear and perceived as more fragile than those of adults.

We want to think that medicine is a unified profession, with physicians, researchers, hospital administrators and others sharing common goals centered around helping and healing patients—but really, it's way more complicated than that. In reality, medicine is frequently a patchwork of turf wars and egos. To be charitable, the medical community is a conglomeration of people who work very hard and maybe don't have time and energy to keep looking at and aiming for the big picture—the mission of healing through the most efficient, up-to-date, patient-centered approaches.

And so, in some ways, Murphy's energy and passion were a detriment when it came to convincing his colleagues to refer patients to him. Traditionally, the medical world encourages diligence and creativity in research, but most physicians, especially those in the academy, treat entrepreneurs as if they are snake-oil salesmen (which, to be fair, in some cases they are). The hierarchy is difficult to challenge. The fact that Murphy was working on a genetics fellowship at Yale was a good start, but it was only a start: he didn't yet have the paper that certified him, or letters beside his name on a plaque on his office wall. He was an MD and eventually became boarded in internal medicine, but he had no official genetics credentials. He was self-taught—which is laudable in some professions, but less so in medicine and science. And he wasn't making a lot of friends in the medical world, people who could actually help him, if they wanted to. At one point or another, the Gene Sherpa had shredded all of his internal medicine colleagues—the very people who might be able to throw him a bone (or patient) or two.

Early in 2009, Murphy received the brochure for the annual meeting of the American College of Physicians, which was to take place in Philadelphia later that year. The American College of Physicians (ACP)—a national organization of internists, with 132,000 members, bills itself on its website as 'Doctors for Adults'—specializing in "the prevention, detection and treatment of illnesses in adults." At first, Murphy was excited. The meeting would be a great opportunity to meet colleagues and get caught up on what was happening in the world of adult medicine, but the more he thumbed through the schedule of scientific sessions and events, the more frustrated he became, not because of what was offered in the program—but what was not.

"Seriously," he read to me from his blog, "they have an entire set of sessions called 'computers in practice'—five goddamn sessions a day devoted to computers in practice, when only 11–15% of physicians have actually adopted the EMRs—electronic medical records. What are the computer topics, in case you are curious?" he asked.

"One: Microsoft Power Point for Beginners. Two: Power Point for Advanced Users. Three: Excel Spreadsheets for Beginners. Four: Getting Started with PDAs. Five: No- and Low-Cost Medical Websites. Six: Useful Medical Applications Using Windows Mobile. I could go on and on, but I tell you, when I read this, I was just about ready to jump out a window.

"If you look closely at the brochure you can see that the meeting is jam-packed with information and events . . . but unfortunately, you will see one huge thing missing . . . That's right, nowhere will you see the word genetics or personalized medicine . . . And that is a crying shame."

How and where, he demanded, will these doctors for adults learn about the future of medicine? "They blew it big-time . . . if they think teaching Power Point is more important than understanding how to interpret a genetic test . . . Where is the Family History for Beginners session? What about the Pharmacogenomics for Beginners? . . . This is a perfect example of why 'Doctors for Adults' are slow to adopt genetics in their practices . . . Because they don't freakin' know it exists . . ."

Murphy was on a rant—which, as I said, is not unusual. And in some ways he was being unfair to the conference organizers, who were trying to ascertain what potential attendees might want to learn (and what would, therefore, entice them to register and attend), and not necessarily what the organizers think their colleagues need to learn. Which is not to say that the American College of Physicians doesn't feel empowered and responsible to continually inform members of ideas and techniques that they feel physicians need to know—or want to know—but it may well be that personalized medicine had not reached that tipping point yet.

Sarah Coombes, a genetic counselor who worked for Steve Murphy for a little more than seven months before switching positions, once tried to explain to her new boss at Sloan Kettering Memorial Hospital exactly what Steve Murphy was trying to accomplish with his personalized medicine practice. But it wasn't easy. Her boss was interested, but his reaction was similar to that of many other doctors she had talked with while working with Murphy: "He jumped to the conclusion that Steve was operating one of these direct-to-consumer, no-physician-involved services like Navigenics or 23andMe—we are going to sell you a test and send you a useless printout—no matter what I told him."

Coombes remembers sitting in front of her boss in his office, repeatedly explaining what Murphy was trying to do. "He wouldn't even let me finish my sentences," she recalls. He had an idea in his head, and he couldn't quite visualize what Murphy was trying to accomplish. "'No, no, no,' I said repeatedly, we were selling a comprehensive medical service, and we were trying to manage a whole person not just related to their link to cancer, but everything across the board that they may benefit from in terms of genetic screening and prevention."

Her boss finally listened, but he didn't think that a personalized medicine private practice could work, and he was totally unenthused about the idea of attempting to accomplish such a feat outside of a major medical center, with its wealth of resources—laboratories, specialists of all varieties and funding for research.

Sarah Coombes's new boss was a renowned oncologist who had been instrumental in discovering the breast cancer gene. He was hardheaded, cranky and egocentric, and he made it clear to me when I talked with him that he thought Murphy was kind of a lightweight—too young and inexperienced.

Murphy was well aware that some of his senior colleagues regarded him as an upstart and opportunist, but he, in turn, looked down on them for being out of touch with the real world—in their "ivy-covered towers." In fact, he was contemplating leaving Yale simply because he thought he was spinning his wheels, wasting time when he could be preaching the personalized medicine gospel and practicing what he was preaching helping his patients—that is, if he had patients. This—the lack of patients—seemed to be a problem he had difficulty confronting. (He did eventually leave Yale and pursue his practice more vigorously.) The fact that his colleagues in research or in private practice were pretty much ignoring his efforts was galling and also humiliating.

But he also understood where they were coming from, especially his brothers in private practice. Physicians are practical people. They will often learn what they need to know only when they need to know it—not before. And this might not be the time for most general practitioners to get onto the genetics/personalized medicine bandwagon. This, of course, has been the ambivalence Murphy has been facing; most physicians feel genetics and personalized medicine are provocative and will someday be essential to understand and to apply—but not now.

And geneticists themselves, mostly hospital-based, characteristically, are slow-movers, thinkers and philosophers, which is the nature of their profession—a different ilk than most other physicians, and with good reason. The American Board of Medical Specialties recognized the American College of Medical Genetics (ACMG) relatively recently, in 1991, as the twenty-fourth primary board of medicine, implying that it represented a unique knowledge base, distinctly different from any other area of medical practice. Unique indeed: all of the other twenty-three specialties are organ based, while genetics is genome based, something that's in every cell and every organ. "In genetics we have maybe 5,000–7,000 rare diseases that we deal with. Nobody can even memorize the entire list, let alone know how to deal with them," says Murphy.

Following the triumph of the HGP you might think the medical world would be teeming with geneticists, or at least would-be geneticists, or even just physicians looking to learn more about this new era of genomic personalization. But in 2009, there were fewer than 1,000 board-certified geneticists in the United States. (By way of comparison, in 2001 there were more than 62,000 board-certified internists.) And even now, the majority of practicing geneticists are pediatricians who have rarely—if at all—treated or prescribed medicine to adult patients in their entire careers.

You might think that this fact alone would compel many more young physicians to enter the field. That, especially when you consider all the new possibilities in the wake of the HGP, medical societies and associations would introduce personalized medicine courses, plan personalized medicine conferences—help colleagues in various subspecialties to achieve a modest level of genetic competence. But in 2008, there were only eighty-three adult internal medicine geneticists in the United States, not even two per state. Two years later, in 2010, there were only a few more—fewer than one-hundred in the entire country.

That people—especially Murphy's colleagues—could not see the handwriting on the wall, recognize the growing evidence that genetics and personalized medicine were the next big things, irritated Murphy to no end. He could not understand why such gifted and intelligent men and women—physicians and scientists—were so resistant. Personalized medicine was not "pie in the sky"; it was real. Was it that his colleagues disagreed with his vision of personalized medicine—or were they simply clueless about genetics or completely distracted by what seemed to them to be more vital concerns in their practices?

Turns out, it was a combination of both.

A 2010 study of 10,000 physicians conducted by the American Medical Association and the pharmacy benefits manager Medco Healthcare Solutions revealed that physicians are well aware that genetic tests can help predict and target more effective treatment in relation to drug therapy for pain, depression, and gastrointestinal and cardiovascular problems. But the tests are rarely ordered not because doctors are unaware that testing can be beneficial, but more so because doctors don't know how to interpret the information provided by the tests. The study showed that only 13% of the physicians surveyed had actually ordered a genetic test over the previous six months—for any reason. And only one in ten of those physicians ordering the tests felt that they knew enough about how to effectively use the information they might receive.

Perhaps he had been naïve, but Murphy initially believed this might be the key to his practice: He and his practice would offer a solution to physicians who knew that genetics could provide important, potentially even life-saving information to their patients, but who were unable, themselves, to become experts. Doctors wouldn't have to turn themselves into geneticists; instead, they could refer their patients to Murphy.

Murphy contended that he knew from the start that the economics would be a challenge; Insurance companies and Medicare reimbursements wouldn't cover the expense of treating patients in the way he wanted to, taking detailed family histories and having long conversations.

"There's no money in it," he said to me once, as if he was uttering a long-running joke and shaking his head, as if he was trapped by circumstance and couldn't really do anything about his predicament, except laugh and soldier onward. He seemed cavalier at times, not really ready to accept the gravity of his situation. Sarah Coombes confirmed that idea. She told me that Murphy seemed paralyzed by the idea that he might actually fail, that his dream of personalized medicine in a day-to-day practice would collapse and that he would be left with nothing but unemployment, bankruptcy and big debt. On the other hand, sometimes situations become so insolvable and out of control and the people involved feel so helpless to intervene or take positive action, to know what to do, after having tried everything they could think of, that all that's left is to laugh, just to exert some emotion and relieve the burden of the ongoing tension.

This was late 2008, more than a year after he had launched his Park Avenue practice. His business, to say the least, was not booming. The plunging stock market was not helping matters, and Murphy was laughing and shaking his head.

"There's no money in the whole damn personalized medicine thing at all! That is what I have come to realize. If only I were an attorney. Maybe I should get a law degree," he said. "If I'm an attorney and I'm prepping for a case I get to bill for every hour. Even though I may not be in court or preparing documents—if I'm actually just thinking about the case, and I'm reading law books to better understand my case, guess what? I can bill." He understands, of course, that attorneys are not billing Medicare—they are collecting fees from the people who hire them or sharing in settlement revenue. "Here I am a doctor—not worrying about briefs and litigation, but caring for someone's life and health, and I can't get paid for researching and thinking, like attorneys, like academics." His feelings of being trapped and doomed eventually surfaced.

"Where do they think I get my knowledge?" he suddenly cried out, blood rushing to his cheeks. "Thin air? Free air? What's going on?"

He took some comfort in knowing that even in major medical centers, where almost all of the geneticists could be found, genetics and genetics programs are not moneymakers. In most states, geneticists—or physicians doing genetics research—are reimbursed by insurance the same amount as an internist conducting a regular routine annual physical examination: approximately $375 in 2009, Murphy told me. While this may seem like a lot of money to folks on a fixed income or hourly wage, it doesn't pay the bills for a physician with a nursing staff, office and other expenses. Procedures like biopsies and blood work are often how physicians make their livings, or how medical centers make profits. Many private-practice physicians have their own laboratories or are tied in with a professional group, pooling resources for maximizing income. But there are few if any "procedures" in genetics.

Insurance companies and Medicare won't reimburse enough, so for his practice to be profitable—or to even pay for itself—Murphy had to find patients willing to pay out of pocket for the work he would do for them. Hence his office location: Park Avenue and 82nd Street—a neighborhood where people, at the time he started, had mounds of disposable income. In fact his first six patients, friends and acquaintances, were all self-pay.

But was it too soon to have made the plunge into personalization? Had he miscalculated the arrival of the tipping point?

Murphy was trying to fuse the intellectual effort of the geneticist with the necessarily fast shoot-from-the-hip action of the general practitioner. But it wasn't working out from the GP point of view, although there were successful interactions between geneticists and other specialists in a growing number of medical centers across the United States.

At the University of North Carolina at Chapel Hill, Jim Evans, professor and director of the Bryson Program in Human Genetics and editor of the *Journal of the American College of Medical Genomics*, oversees a program that tries to bridge the gap between physicians and geneticists, and to make it easier for patients to be connected to geneticists for family histories. Evans is foty-five, short yet gangly, with a sharp nose, a high forehead and a folksy, Jimmy Stewart drawl. He has a staff of genetic counselors who see patients already in the hospital for evaluation or treatment of other diseases. "What we're doing here," Evans explained, "is what I call the 'deployment model.' We have a team of genetic counselors who go out to other clinics in the medical center—ophthalmology, cardiology, nephrology, dermatology, hematology and, like today, oncology—and work with the physicians." In many ways, Evans's staff is networking, looking for new customers who can benefit from genetic testing. In most medical centers, the geneticist is an outsider, but Evans—who began his career in private practice—is, like Murphy, aggressively attempting to bring together doctors from all different subspecialties.

In addition to conducting family histories and counseling patients, Evans and his corps of genetic counselors also attend the specialty conferences—when all of the attending doctors, the residents and nurses meet to discuss the patients, examine X-rays, debate diagnosis and agree on treatment plans. After a while, the counselors are included in the conversation. "Or," said Evans, "when they are discussing the patient, the counselor can pipe up and say, 'Well, this is exactly the kind of patient we need to consider in genetics, so we'll go ahead and see them and then we'll report back to you what we find out.' It becomes a multidisciplinary approach, and that way it's a patient-centric approach and you're helping the patient, but what you're also doing, I think, real importantly, is you're teaching those clinicians about the genetic aspects that are germane and practical for them to know."

Also like Murphy, Evans is somewhat fanatical about genetics. I once asked him: "Why did you go into genetics? What makes it so special?"

Evans's face immediately lit up—he was glowing!—and he nearly screamed, "Oh, because it is the coolest thing I can imagine!" He was suddenly very excited. "It is beautiful," he added, waxing as if in a trance. "It is beautiful in the same sense that Newton's Laws of motion are beautiful—simple ideas which explain a vast amount of seemingly impenetrable, complex observations. The fall of an apple, the orbit of the moon around the sun, is directly analogous to the way genetics explains much of that part of biology that seems chaotic and unapproachable." Evans pointed to a poem by Thomas Hardy, "Heredity," in

a frame on his wall. He starts all of his medical school courses, he said, by
reading the poem aloud.

> I am the family face;
> Flesh perishes, I live on,
> Projecting trait and trace
> Through time to times anon,
> And leaping from place to place
> Over oblivion.
>
> The years-heired feature that can
> In curve and voice and eye
> Despise the human span
> Of durance—that is I;
> The eternal thing in man,
> That heeds no call to die.

"Genetics is simple and it is elegant," Evans said. "And yet, its explanatory
power is tremendous. It says something very fundamental about who we are:
the product of our environment and, to an undeniable extent, a product of our
genes." He turned to look at his computer, which revealed an ongoing montage
of his family photographs. "How happy we are, how sad, our levels of sociality,
of religiosity—these are all concepts rooted in our genes."

Evans compared the principles of genetics with an understanding of evolution:
"In both evolution and genetics, we have a very simple concept that explains an
unfathomable amount of information about the world around us—so logical
and amazing, especially when you suddenly see how it all comes together so
beautifully."

Does he actually walk down the street and think stuff like this, that genetics
is cool and beautiful? Such idealism in this day and age is rather rare—very
different from, say, surgeons, who typically describe their work using dramatic
terms like "critical" or "harrowing," or family practice physicians who say their
work is "satisfying" or "helpful" or "crucial."

"Yeah! Yeah!" Evans drawled, his voice skyrocketing upward. "I do! I do!" He
leaned forward, as if to emphasize his sincerity. "I will frequently look at a tree and
it sometimes will strike me forcibly that that tree uses the same genetic code as I

do—in every living cell of that pine tree there is DNA, which is transcribed and translated in the same way we are. It is a commonality with the rest of the universe that is really quite striking. We are related to that tree, not in a metaphorical sense, but in a *literal* sense." He hurried on, waving his arms. "You go back to your parents'-parents'-parents'-parents and go back to that tree's parents'-parents'-parents'-parents, go back all the way down the line . . . ," he paused. His eyes were gleaming, and his cheeks flushed. "And guess what! They will fuse!" Again he paused, and then whispered, shaking his head: "Genetics! It is stunning."

CHAPTER 6:
A LACK OF RESPECT

Evans and Murphy are in the small minority of physicians who love and promote genetics. The fact that there are few of them is not surprising. In a culture where "doers" are responsible for most of the revenue, thinkers usually get short shrift. By "doers" I mean surgeons or other physicians that require procedures that are mostly expensive and often repetitious, if not overprescribed. But the very act of considering genetics in the mix demands caution, contemplation and conversation—anathema in many healthcare centers. As a prominent transplant surgeon stated in relation to a conversation about a patient's diagnosis: "I don't have time to talk about it; I am too busy saving lives."

This attitude makes for an uphill battle in the genetics world and unfortunately seems to create an atmosphere of insecurity and resentment in the genetics field, especially in clinical settings. Despite the HGP and the oft-discussed oncoming era of personalized medicine, even the most committed geneticists are unsure of their futures.

Bruce Korf is a tall, soft-spoken, geeky-looking guy with a long neck, a pointed nose, sloping shoulders and slicked-back, graying hair. He left Harvard in 2003, where he had been an attending physician for twenty years, to move to Alabama because, in part, of Harvard's reluctance to introduce full-fledged genetics training as part of the medical curriculum. Korf has been able to do that in Birmingham.

We had a long conversation one morning in his office about the rising prospects and pitfalls of the field of genetics. But when I asked him about the future prospects of personalized medicine, which is a more comprehensive subject than genetics, especially in relation to his very large group of genetics residents and fellows—one of the largest in the United States—he didn't answer, at least not right away.

He looked at me for a moment, then he said, "It depends on what you mean by personalized medicine." He paused again, and then continued. "I think," said Korf, "that you will probably find that our residents, if you were to ask that question, might not even know what you were asking. Their days are not filled with 'How do I deal with pharmacogenomics?' 'How do I counsel people based on a family history of diabetes and hypertension?'—the kind of things you hear about when you discuss personalized medicine. That is barely on their radar screen on a day-to-day basis. I don't want you to think that personalized medicine is the life's blood of what residents think about every day. We certainly do talk about it. It is part of their training, but not like the day-to-day experience they have."

This may be true in some medical centers, but in my experience, I have discovered that young physicians (residents, interns, even med students) are much more aware of the term and interested in it than are many of their teachers and supervisors. This has been a problem in the medical community—a generation gap between the "Here's how I learned medicine, so that is how you should learn medicine, also" group of traditionalists who control the substance of medical education at the moment, and the young people, like Murphy, who want to learn and apply new ideas and practices.

I once interviewed a group of genetics fellows and residents at a major medical center. Although they were very comfortable defining and discussing "personalized medicine," they were quite frustrated because they sometimes felt marginalized— not necessarily unaccepted as much as ignored—and not on the radar of senior colleagues in other subspecialties. They were referring to the atmosphere not only in their own medical center, but also in medical circles in the United States in general.

Residents and fellows in genetics have chosen genetics as a career direction, so they are well educated in their specialty, but for medical students and other residents there are few genetics training options. Genetics is touched upon when appropriate but not focused on in most medical schools, as of yet. Physicians in training are expected to somehow absorb genetic information and knowledge amorphously as they progress—a reality that can be quite detrimental to patients, these residents told me. They traded war stories.

One resident complained that in certain cases infants who seemed to be suffering from failure-to-thrive issues were given "g" tubes—gastrointestinal feeding tubes to bulk up their weight and nutrition—because genetic testing is too often an afterthought. Genetic testing might show that children are small because of inherent genetic conditions, but that their growth is normal considering those conditions. In such cases, "g" tubes could be detrimental.

Sometimes physicians who are not geneticists diagnose genetic syndromes without seeking help or confirmation from a geneticist. This tendency can also cause difficulties. One resident recalled a pregnant woman who had come to the hospital for a prenatal ultrasound. She had eye problems which her ophthalmologist had said were caused by a genetic syndrome, Peters plus, which is characterized by short stature, developmental delay and eye abnormalities. The resident was part of the team that followed the mom in the prenatal ultrasound clinic. Team members could see in the ultrasounds that the fetus was smaller than normal for its gestational age, which was not unexpected if the baby also had Peters plus. The resident was on call the day the baby was born. "The baby came out," said the resident, "with no eyes." The technical term for the condition is anophthalmia.

A subsequent genetics consult and a family history uncovered previously unknown information—and the fact that Peters plus was not an accurate diagnosis. The father, like the mother, suffered from serious eye abnormalities and, perhaps even more telling, the father and mother were reportedly first cousins. Even with all of this information, they could not determine the exact diagnosis—why the child was born with anophthalmia—but had a geneticist been called in at the outset, he or she would have undoubtedly discovered that the original diagnosis was incorrect. And doctors would have been able to prepare the parents more realistically for the surprise of having a child born with no eyes.

A couple of the residents around the table that day began discussing a patient who became pregnant through sperm donation. All went well for mother and babies—she had twins—until a year later, when she received a letter from the sperm bank informing her that the donor was a carrier of a debilitating and incurable neuromuscular disease. Her reproductive endocrinologist assured her that she had nothing to worry about—it takes two carriers in this instance to affect a child—and ordered a test. Turned out the mother was a carrier. As in the situation of the child with no eyes, neither the endocrinologist nor the geneticist could have made a difference, medically. But the doctor made matters worse by not referring the mother to a geneticist who would have recognized the potential seriousness of the problem and walked her through the test and its range of outcomes. A major role for the geneticist, or perhaps even more for the genetic counselors who work side by side with the geneticist, is to provide patients with information—and then to help them make decisions based on that information.

But doctors are also often hesitant to refer their patients to geneticists because they believe that the geneticist will sidetrack or upset the patient or the family or talk the patient to death, especially when it is time to take action—for example, to opt for radical surgery or a trial medication. "Many subspecialists think that we worry their patients too much," said a geneticist at Harvard. "I heard one of the cardiologists say to a genetics resident, 'I just don't want you to upset my patient.' Well, my response to that is that the parents already know that their child has a birth defect or whatever the problem is, and all we would do is try to clarify what the cause of the problem was—to help them understand. I think they are already plenty worried."

Geneticists are also known to take up a lot of valuable time, a practice that does not serve the medical profession too well, even though the geneticist begins his or her work by talking with patients—which is good, and important—and collecting a great deal of personal information about their lives and families. And this is just to get the ball rolling. There are few cut-and-dried answers when a physician is sorting through an array of 5,000 possible diseases and countless possible genetic mutations. After the family history, which, as Murphy has pointed out, is an ongoing conversation, a geneticist will go online or consult textbooks for more research, reach out to colleagues and devote time to contemplation and thought. Immediate action is unusual.

A recent study conducted by the Department of Medical Genetics at the Marshfield Clinic in Wisconsin documented the time-intensive nature of the profession. Over a ten-week period during clinics, both geneticists and genetic counselors recorded their time in fifteen-minute increments using an electronic timer. For this study, on the average, physicians logged 54.1 hours and counselors 43.5 hours per week, with physicians devoting about half their time and counselors three quarters of their time to patient care or other patient-related activities. Total patient time averaged seven hours for a new patient and about 3.5 hours for follow-up work. Unfortunately, however, only 15% of the patient care time was billable, under the current reimbursement system.

Although she is not disputing the time it takes to see patients, as documented in the Marshfield study, Mira Irons, Director of the Genetics Residency program and Genetics Fellowship training programs at Harvard Medical School, suggests that taking seven hours to see a patient, during a time when the need for clinical genetics is expanding and the number of geneticists entering the field is decreasing, is, to put it bluntly, "absurd." At the other end of the spectrum, consumer-driven screening companies offer what seems to be an easy and inexpensive alternative to the lengthy interview process—but might not offer quite enough information to help patients. Certainly many doctors, as Sarah Coombes's new boss indicated, were legitimately appalled by this discounted shortcut method of diagnosis.

Another complication is that doctors, especially internists, are used to having "yes" and "no" answers—positive and negative results from blood tests. But with genetic testing almost nothing is that clear; all genetic tests require a qualifying discussion. Just because you identify a mutation doesn't mean that you have really confirmed that condition. Those "qualifying discussions" are often serious barriers. Doctors believe, rightly, that they are not adequately reimbursed for such conversations, and so they are cautious and sometimes reluctant and resentful, not to mention ill equipped, to discuss genetic links to cancer and other diseases. Murphy is a rare breed, a private practice doctor willing to accept the authorized reimbursement for a forty-five-minute talking time. Most patient-physicians interactions take place in an average of twelve-minute sessions.

The residents I talked with were concerned about their futures. If patients can't or won't go to geneticists, and if their GPs won't refer them, then what of their career goals and income potential? Dermatology would be a lot cleaner and considerably more profitable, as Steve Murphy was finding out.

Even Bruce Korf concedes: "I don't think you could argue that the average graduate from medical school today is prepared to use genetic testing for risk assessment and choice of medication in disease stratification: the kind of things that personalized medicine is usually assumed to include. But at this moment, personalized medicine is not practiced to a large degree in this country. And there's the dilemma: training people not for what you can do right now, but for what you're going to be able to do a bit downstream, doesn't make a lot of sense."

Korf does not know Steve Murphy, but he offers an example relevant to Murphy's Park Avenue experiment. "It reminds me a little bit like something my father did, which was to set up a store to sell televisions in 1952. It didn't last very long as a business. And you say to yourself, 'Wow, they're really in on the ground floor of something that's going to be revolutionary,' and it was. But there is such a thing as being in on it a little too early—which is what happened to my dad."

"Some of my best friends tell me I'm wasting my time or I'm ahead of the time—or that I am just plain crazy," Murphy told me. "I tell them, 'No, I'm not crazy. I am obsessed—and I won't be deterred.'"

CHAPTER 7:
INSPIRATION—
AND FRUSTRATION

The marketers Steve Murphy had engaged recommended a multifaceted plan of action: get in better contact with private practice physicians and tell them what he could do; and identify those physicians most likely to refer. Probably this would be oncologists, because the first entrance to personalized medicine at that moment—and still today—was breast and ovarian cancers. Families of women (and men) diagnosed with breast cancer might want to know if they have the *BRCA* gene.

Murphy and his genetic counselor Sarah Coombes started to reach out to these physicians, mostly around the Greenwich area, where his contacts were strong, rather than in New York. "We immediately identified tremendous barriers," he said. "Not just 'What do you do in personalized medicine?' but also 'What good is it—how can it help my patients?' 'What about genetic discrimination?' 'Isn't this too expensive?' On and on."

Murphy, Coombes, and Adam Messenger, a colleague at Greenwich Hospital who hoped one day to join Murphy's practice full-time, also went on the road, explaining personalized medicine to anyone who would listen. "We went to conferences, did lunches, doctor visits. And it worked!" Murphy said, laughing. "We had sixty to seventy referrals before we knew it.

"But in fact," he added, "we didn't know it."

This was perhaps the most frustrating result of his efforts back then: he had some of the doctors on board, finally, and, as it turned out, temporarily. "Because here was a second roadblock—one we hadn't foreseen. The docs would say to their patients, 'I want you to see Dr. Murphy.' But patients weren't calling us. They weren't picking up the phone. The patients weren't listening." The economy certainly had a lot to do with patients' reluctance to follow their doctor's recommendations and see a geneticist. And the fear of genetic discrimination was an equally powerful reason why patients were hesitant to reach out to Murphy.

That day in New York when Murphy and I were on our way to do the family history and blood test, the day we ran into my friend on the street, Murphy received a series of phone calls from the doctor who had referred a patient. It turned out that the patient was having second thoughts about her consultation with Murphy because she was afraid that confidential information about her would not be protected by the company doing the test, Myriad Genetics and Laboratory.

Murphy assured the physician that Myriad maintains confidentiality, sharing information with no one except the physician requesting the blood work, the referring physician (if there is one) and the patient. But the patient wanted assurances from Myriad, and refused to see Murphy—and the referring physician refused to allow Murphy to approach the patient—until Murphy had a conversation with a Myriad official and obtained the necessary assurances. When Murphy contacted his representative at Myriad, she was unavailable. Murphy was frustrated and perplexed. His outward cool and confidence seemed somewhat shaken. All through our conversation, his cell phone would ring with additional questions from the referring physician and Murphy would be back on the phone, leaving increasingly anxious voice-mail messages at Myriad.

Obviously, these complications did not occur every day—and he knew when the Genetic Information Nondiscrimination Act (GINA) was signed into law, which it was, eventually, in 2008, that patients' apprehension about being outed would be less intense. But neither, alas, did Murphy have referrals every day—or every week, for that matter—and he wanted to make the most of the opportunity so that the referring physician would refer again and not consider it too troublesome to do so. Murphy and I spent a discouraging early afternoon together with him attempting to sound upbeat about the future of personalized medicine, while at the same time confronting an obstacle to the most basic and anchoring element of the entire idea.

Murphy eventually worked out the problem with the patient that day. The Myriad representative returned his phone call, gave him adequate assurances (which, of course, he already knew) and offered to telephone the referring doctor directly, if the problem persisted. And so Murphy was permitted to follow through and conduct the family history, but his frustration was palpable.

That day, in order to do a family history, just to satisfy the referring doctor, he had canceled a scheduled visit to Yale, where he was seeing patients—and now his whole day was falling apart.

"This ethics question, I mean the divulging or concealing of genetic information, is just at the tip of the iceberg," he said. "Just wait!" This was certainly true, I would discover as my research continued. The more we attempt to integrate personalized medicine and genetic information into the healthcare system, the more roadblocks and hurdles will appear—and not so easily disappear without involving lawyers, hospital administrators and doctors and their patients.

But in some ways Murphy's struggle to see his patient and the way in which his day had collapsed around him, and even all of the ethical and legal difficulties he was forced to confront, didn't matter in the end. Steve Murphy was a true believer in genetics and in his vision, and he insisted, each time I asked him, almost tauntingly, if he was ready to give up and return to a traditional medical practice, that nothing would change him because he had been a true believer even before the sequencing of the genome had taken place.

"The first time I heard the word 'genetics,' I was eight years old," he remembered. "I was watching one of those *GI Joe* episodes on TV, and in this particular episode they were trying to figure out how to create this super villain. They went to all the tombs of all of these dead evil people, Genghis Khan, Hitler, whoever, and they were drawing DNA out of these people to create the super villain, and GI Joe was fighting them and trying to keep them out of these tombs from getting the super-villain DNA. They took DNA samples from a collection of the meanest people they could find in the world. But then GI Joe cloned a second super villain badder than the first super villain in order to destroy him. I will always remember that—my first introduction to DNA. I thought, *this was so cool*."

A more realistic and equally persuasive experience years later while he was in medical school at New York Medical College (he earned his undergraduate degree at Penn State) accelerated Murphy's interest to full-blown obsession. "A patient, a young boy, came into the hospital with burning and tingling in his hands," he explained. "Painful. It got worse in warm weather." The boy had been in the hospital for two weeks, and no one could figure out what was going on. "Test after test," said Murphy. "And nothing. No information and no relief for this boy."

Murphy cannot now remember why he became so concerned with this boy—there were many needy patients in the hospital, as always—except to say that he did not like the idea of not knowing what was wrong. He enjoyed the challenges of research and had considered pursuing a PhD, but more than anything, he had come to the medical world, decided to be a doctor, in order to interact with people in trouble—sick and suffering—and help them. "But you can't help a patient, at least in the long run, and you can't really treat, without a diagnosis," he said.

"I went to see a friend, a neurology resident at Westchester [NY] Hospital and I said to him, 'I have this patient'—I described the symptoms—'can you help me out?'" His friend was too busy to dig into the problem with him, but Murphy's description of the boy immediately rang a bell, and he directed Murphy to the residents' room to retrieve an article, newly published in the *New England Journal of Medicine* (NEJM), about painful peripheral neuropathies. Painful peripheral neuropathies are basically related to damaged nerve systems. The article included a chart isolating age groups and symptoms with connections to specific neuropathies that induce pain. The article told Murphy everything he needed to know. He had a diagnosis. "Bingo! There it was! A genetic condition—a mutation!" he announced. "Fabry Disease."

"It was so obvious," he said, smiling and shrugging, "in retrospect." He went to the medical library at Mt. Sinai and read everything he could about Fabry Disease. Murphy learned that people suffering from Fabry Disease had families with histories of stroke, sudden cardiac death, cardiomyopathy and kidney failure. The mutated gene that causes Fabry is carried on a mother's X chromosome, and the disease is more common in males than in females. Murphy returned to see the boy, conducted an informal family history and found almost identical similarities between the patient's history and the symptoms of Fabry Disease.

The next day, Steve Murphy listened as the intern assigned to the patient presented the case at chairman's rounds and made a diagnosis—reflex sympathetic dystrophy. This is a condition of burning pain, stiffness, swelling, and discoloration of the hand, so it wasn't really a bad diagnosis, Murphy said. "But it didn't sound exactly right, as it turned out, which is exactly what the chairman of the department remarked, after he listened to the intern. 'Okay, possible. But I think it is something else.'"

Murphy set the scene; he remembered that day, perhaps more than any other day in his medical training, because it gave him an irreversible direction: The chairman was sitting at a conference table with some of the other "attendings"—

faculty-level doctors. The interns sat in a row behind the attendings. Murphy was sitting with the other medical students, "in the outer circle, like it's the peanut gallery," Murphy remembered. He stood up and announced, "I know what it is! It's Fabry Disease!" Then he listed all of the reasons why he thought it was Fabry Disease. When he finished, no one said anything. Silence.

"I am thinking, 'This is the end of my career'—I mean, I must be making no sense at all. So I slink back in my chair, sit and wait. And then the chairman goes: 'Okay, maybe you're right. Call the geneticist.' I make the call later, get the guy on the phone and quickly describe the case. And he says—takes him two seconds, fast!—'Your patient has Fabry Disease.'

"And suddenly that was it for me," said Murphy, waving his hands and raising his voice. He was glowing with excitement. "What a fantastic field, I thought. The guy, this doctor—a *geneticist*—takes bits and pieces of information gathered from the simple details of a family history from a med student—just the stuff I had put together quickly—and out comes a diagnosis. In two seconds! What a way to help people! What a way to think!" The clarity and logic of it all astounded him. "I knew that I had to be a part of this world."

After medical school, Murphy went to Mt. Sinai Medical Center in New York, perhaps the best place in the world at the time for pediatrics and genetics, but after two years he had had enough of "peeds." He decided he wanted to practice internal medicine so he moved into the Yale system, which placed him at Greenwich Hospital. He actually almost decided to decline the Greenwich offer because his wife, Dana, whom he had met and married in medical school, was a radiology resident at Columbia. Eventually Dana decided to leave radiology and transfer into adult internal medicine, like her husband, serving a residency at Greenwich Hospital. "So we have a lot to talk about, every day," Murphy said—not only medicine, but also their young child, a two-year-old. But his family responsibilities were about to change. The next time I saw him at Greenwich Hospital, a few weeks later, he told me his "from bad to good" story.

He was supposed to drive Dana to work that morning, but he was procrastinating, so she became annoyed and left the house without him. "But she slipped on the ice while walking to our car." He took her to the ER. But talk about bad to good: "Turns out she broke her elbow," Murphy said. "That's the bad news—which precipitated an exam which led to the good news. She's pregnant with our second child!"

I asked if he was nervous, considering the insecurity of his practice. "I'm delighted; I'm excited—no reason to wait until we get old," he said, "to have a second child and continue to build our family. But that means I am going to have to make some decisions rather quickly." He was referring to whether he should be reevaluating his direction and taking advantage of more lucrative job opportunities, like the one in concierge medicine. Dana, it should be said, does not have as much enthusiasm for personalized medicine as her husband, Murphy told me. But Murphy's enthusiasm makes up for the both of them—plus half the population of Greenwich.

Before launching his practice, Steve Murphy made up his mind to practice what he preached and start with his own family history as "Patient Zero"—a test case. First, Murphy met with a genetic counselor and outlined his history as he remembered it. Next, Murphy's parents got involved. His mother was interviewed, and then she researched her own mother's medical history. Murphy's grandmother had died of metastatic breast cancer. His mother reached out to an aunt who had early-onset breast cancer, to gather her medical records and identify her diagnosis.

There is, however, an unavoidable gap in Murphy's family history. His whole name is Steven Andrew Rivera Murphy. His biological father, born in Puerto Rico, was a Rivera who abandoned the family when Steve was young. His stepfather, a farm worker, was a Murphy. "Raised me from five years old on and really helped me out through childhood, guided me and mentored me and so I took the name Murphy but I kept the name Rivera."

So the family history process went well, as far as it could go. And yet Murphy knew that taking one family history was a good start—but not nearly what he wanted for his practice or what he knew the medical world needed.

"To really make personalized medicine personalized, you have to follow patients for the rest of their lives," he said. "You start when they are born—which is the way of the future—and one doctor or group of doctors should follow you and your family for a lifetime. Patients should be regularly monitored. Your family may be fine this week, but next week, God forbid, your youngest sister may suddenly be discovered suffering with cancer and maybe she's only forty years old. That could make other members of the family change how they live or what they intend to do about their own family or lifestyles. Or your father who's fifty-two may have dropped dead from a heart attack." Your family history is not really history like you learn in school; it is dynamic and ever evolving. Said Murphy, "If I take your family history once and call it a day, walk away, send a bill, then truly, I've done you a disservice."

In some ways it could be said that Murphy's obsession had done his family a great disservice, as well. In addition to his medical loans for school, which totalled $250,000, Murphy had borrowed $200,000 to start his practice—and another $100,000 from his mother to supplement his start-up expenses. In his early thirties, he was beginning his adult life burdened by debt. It is ironic that family and history were the anchoring elements of Steve Murphy's practice. For if it wasn't for a tragic event in the history of his own family—one that was directly related to the medical world—he would have been unable to launch his practice and fulfill his dream.

"My mother suffered from mistreatment from a doctor," he explained. "She has had twenty surgeries on her back since she was a teenager and multiple spinal fusions that caused gross infections." Part of the money he had invested came from a malpractice award—gross negligence on the part of his mother's doctor. "My parents [his mother and stepfather] have their hopes on me," said Murphy. "High hopes. They put their money on my dream of a personalized medicine practice, hoping for the security and the long-term care they might have gotten from the money. Now they will need to get the money back. That is a tremendous amount of responsibility—to prove that personalized medicine is the way of the future and to fulfill my obligation to my parents. For both reasons, I feel the pressure every moment I am awake."

CHAPTER 8:
EXPLOITATION

While most physicians in private practice were not yet ready to acknowledge the brave new world that Bill Clinton and Steve Murphy anticipated, people outside of the healthcare community began to recognize the potential impact of the HGP beyond the boundaries of science and healthcare. Some of the fancier department stores jumped on the genetics bandwagon, adding promotions and products that generated a buzz, and profits. Cheek-swabbing stations were set up at their cosmetics counters, and marketing materials promised women all the beauty secrets that the HGP had to offer—whatever those were. Surely Collins and Venter had not given cosmetics a serious thought, but many others devised various profitable applications. A faddish "nutraceuticals" industry sprung up, promising to use genomics to analyze how the customer metabolized food and, interestingly enough, what kind of skin products she should use. But these early companies could not offer anything like a full genomic screening. Instead, they would test one or two genes. The genetic test was just the bait; the profits came from selling supplements or skin creams that were supposedly tailored to the customer's genotype.

Of course, reputable companies also sold genetic tests directly to patients. But the legit services often did not turn a profit, and many customers wanted more than just a lab result. They craved a perfume, a cream in a midnight-blue bottle or a jar full of miracle pills—something, anything, to make their genetic adventure more tangible. A piece of the HGP they could hold.

The market quickly mushroomed. Start-up genetics companies emerged all over the country, many of them based in living rooms and basements. The market became so chaotic that in 2006 the United States Senate decided to clean up the netherworld of direct-to-consumer DNA testing. Government investigators posed as consumers, sending out cheek swabs to several companies. Not surprisingly, every company diagnosed the same patient differently—and many of them recommended that the patient buy exorbitantly priced, "personalized" nutritional supplements. The chairman of a 2006 Senate hearing on home DNA testing, Gordon H. Smith, called these tests "modern-day snake oil." This scamming continues to the present day and federal investigators continue to pursue and penalize violators.

Though the market then was crowded with scammers, a few entrepreneurs dreamed of offering an entirely different kind of service. These companies—Navigenics, 23andMe and a few others—hoped to be able to give customers some small glimpse of their destinies. Customers would log in to websites that explained (in exhaustive and sometimes wonky detail) what their results—which were very limited, compared to whole genome screening—meant. As new medical studies became available, customers would learn ever more about the implications of their own genetic codes.

Would customers pay upward of a thousand dollars for a service that offered nuanced medical information, rather than magic pills? In 2007, as Steve Murphy was pounding the Park Avenue pavements looking for patients, it seemed they might—although not to Murphy.

That was the year that the very aged James Watson shuffled up onto stage and blinked as flashbulbs popped around him. He held up two DVDs containing the entire code of his genome, all of the genes that design and maintain his body. According to the fanfare surrounding this event, Watson had become the first person to hold his own genome in his hand. The achievement was enormous: it had cost a million dollars and taken two months to read all of Watson's genes. A company called 454 Life Sciences had donated this service to Watson, in hopes of creating buzz about its new gene-sequencing technology. Its executives predicted that soon a more affordable entire-genome sequence might become part of a patient's general workup.

The company had picked Watson because, as the surviving member of the team that discovered the double helix, he had become a kind of walking symbol for DNA. That day onstage, he looked sharp for a septuagenarian. Two tufts of white hair exploded from his bald head; he wore a white suit jacket and matching pants that gave him a Gatsby-ish glow. And he played his part perfectly: after shaking hands all around, he brandished the DVDs and hurried away, without offending anyone.

Of course, most of Watson's health story had already been told. After all, if he'd made it to age seventy-nine, he probably did not have the genes that would doom him to Huntington's disease or cystic fibrosis. There was very little in his genes that could predict his future, since he had relatively little future left. And Watson made it clear he didn't want to know about the risks that did face him: he'd asked the company to delete information about one of the genes that indicates a propensity to Alzheimer's disease.

In fact, the gene in question—the *APOE-ε4*—couldn't predict, definitively, whether he would ever suffer from Alzheimer's. It could really only change the way he and his doctors thought about his odds. And that's the danger of genes: it's tempting to read too much into them, to begin to believe in high-tech jinxes and curses. Even Watson, it transpired, was vulnerable to this and harbored a number of crazy ideas about the new technology; in remarks made a few months later, he insisted that white people are smarter than black people and predicted the discovery of genes responsible for creating differences in human intelligence.

In 2008, genetics-testing companies could still imagine they had a huge market to conquer: every American was a potential customer, even if it was not clear why the average man or woman *needed* a printout of his or her genome. This, perhaps, explains the lavish, DNA-related parties of that year, events where models roamed like gazelles among jocks and rich old men in pinstripe suits. Genetic data was the new must-have accessory—or so the publicity agents said.

Navigenics set up a temporary boutique in SoHo to sell its $2,500 test kits just down the street from the showrooms of designers Helmut Lang and Anna Sui. During New York's Fashion Week that year, media mogul Barry Diller welcomed the crowd at a 23andMe party, which he compared to a "seventies sex extravaganza." Lubricated by cocktails, attendees could repair to a "spit lounge" to fill vials and chatter about their earwax and other genetically determined traits.

Meanwhile, that year an online dating service dangled the promise of better loving through genetics. The cofounder of ScientificMatch.com, Eric Holzle, had experienced his eureka moment while watching a documentary about the "sweaty T-shirt experiment." According to that study, women preferred the stench of men with immune systems different than their own; this led, naturally, to the assumption that a pair of lovers with different types of immune systems would have totally hot sex (and down the line, perhaps, robust and healthy offspring). Holzle designed an entire service around that idea, and in 2008, his company offered memberships for about $2,000 that included the test necessary to sort daters into immune-system categories. ScientificMatch.com is still in business, as of this writing, and the $2,000 price tag remains in effect.

And yet, amid all the hype and silliness—the "spit parties," the genetic dating services, the personalized face creams—genetic testing was growing up. The best companies found ways to turn a genetic reading into more than just a horoscope. They developed sophisticated websites that educated customers in all the gray areas surrounding most genetic results. And their highly educated clientele began asking each other questions and sharing information.

Genetic testing 2.0 may offer very different services from those available to consumers today. Companies will likely give out genetic tests for free; in exchange, they will ask customers to share information about their genes and health history; they will then be able to sell this data to Big Pharma—the giant pharmaceutical companies—or use it to generate their own medical insights.

Genetic testing is part of a radical new trend in medicine, one in which consumers expect to interact directly with their own bodies, collecting and storing information themselves.

It's helpful to remember how new this idea really is; as recently as the 1960s, only a handful of Americans had ever used a medical test at home. The women's movement changed all that: women who felt they could not trust their doctors (almost all of whom were male) looked elsewhere for rape counseling, birth control and sometimes abortions.

It was abortions, in particular, that forced many patients to become their own doctors or to pursue home treatments. Before 1973, when the procedure was still illegal, groups like Chicago Women's Liberation Union operated through a system of Xeroxed flyers and sub-rosa phone calls. Desperate women dialed numbers they had found on creased sheets of paper; the phone numbers changed often and left the would-be patient hanging on a disconnected line. Those who managed to get an answer would hear the following message: "Hello, this is Jane from Women's Liberation. Leave your name and number and speak slowly and clearly. Someone will return your call. If you do not hear from us in two or three days, call us back." The word "Jane" was a code—it meant abortion.

Linnea Johnson, one of the members of the Jane collective, remembers how urgently she wanted to do "something real" in 1970. Only twenty-three years old, she'd already divorced the husband who'd mistreated her, and given herself an abortion. Her story (which has been archived by the Chicago Women's Liberation Union) reveals a lot about what life was like before medical testing could be done in the home.

In 1970, Johnson attended a National Organization of Women meeting where the group of activists sat around plotting to throw a cocktail party for advertising executives. Johnson turned to the activist next to her at the meeting and asked, "Is there anything real going on in Chicago for women? This cocktail party stuff is ridiculous."

Soon, Johnson was shuttling around to secret locations to help perform medical procedures. Often, a man in a white coat presided, someone with a bit of conventional medical training. But the Janes did most of the work. Women like Johnson handled the counseling, helping women to understand what would be involved in the secret abortion. Johnson remembers that she would invite clients over in the evening, after her two children had fallen asleep. In front of a fire, with a plate of cookies, Johnson would take down the stranger's medical history and would explain the procedure. She would show the woman a newsprint version of diagrams of the cervix in *Our Bodies, Ourselves* (the information had yet to be published in book form). She'd hand the woman a speculum.

The Jane movement became famous for its illegal activities, but the group also quietly pioneered a new kind of medical testing: the Chicago collective administered medical tests. In the early 1970s, it was possible to order a rudimentary lab kit that included everything necessary for a pregnancy test. No one—except the Janes and a few other feminist groups—seemed to realize that this lab kit represented a little revolution: it could easily be used by a woman at home, in privacy.

The Janes also performed even more complicated medical tests on their own. The Pap test, for instance, required some actual lab work. After swabbing the patient's cervix, Johnson remembered later, "We placed the cells . . . on a glass slide labeled with her name and the date; [we] used fixative and later sent that slide [to a lab] . . . The lab charged us about a dollar per slide for their reading and report." Johnson found this test the most satisfying, because it allowed her to save lives. It was the Pap test, maybe more than anything else, that convinced her that the tools of medicine should be liberated from the doctors. According to Johnson, "The Pap test is no more difficult to do [and] little more invasive or complex than flossing a tooth."

That was perhaps an exaggeration. However, the pregnancy test *was* easy enough for women to use on their own. Feminist groups around the country began helping women obtain the necessary equipment to perform two-hour tests. When *Our Bodies, Ourselves* finally appeared in book form in 1973, it urged women to collect their own urine samples and send them to a lab in North Carolina.

The pharmaceutical industry took note. In 1976, several companies applied to the FDA to sell home pregnancy test kits and won approval. Of course, in order to make the products a success, pharmaceutical companies would have to change cultural norms, convincing women to feel no shame when they walked up to the drugstore counter with a test in hand. As scholar Sarah Abigail Leavitt notes, conservative voices were loud in their tsk-tsking of the home tests. But the pharmaceutical companies returned fire with a blast of advertisements, insisting that women—married or not—had the right to "a private little revolution."

The HIV test kit, when it appeared, faced more vigorous opposition. In 1988, several companies were readying kits that would have required the consumer to collect his or her own blood sample and send it into a lab for discreet testing. The FDA sent stern letters warning companies that these tests could be sold only to medical professionals. Back then, HIV infection amounted to a death sentence, and experts felt that the grim news should be delivered by counselors. It wasn't until 1996 that the FDA opened up the market to do-it-yourself tests for HIV.

By that time, the home-testing revolution had begun in earnest, with drugstores offering entire aisles full of diagnostic equipment, from blood-pressure monitors to a test for urinary-tract infections. With the growth of the Internet, hundreds of products have turned into thousands. Today, in the privacy of your own bathroom, you can diagnose everything from a yeast infection to chicken-feather allergy to a Vitamin D deficiency. It's even legal to test *other* people's bodies; parents can use a commercial drug test to find whether their kids are snorting coke or smoking pot.

Unfortunately, few researchers have bothered to study whether home testing actually does us any good. A medical journal reported in 2006 that there exists almost no data on the effect of this kind of self-monitoring. "An estimation of the clinical or public health impact of any home testing method is nearly pure guesswork at this time," the authors of the study concluded.

So in the end, little can be said about do-it-yourself testing besides, "We don't know." We don't know how people react to their rapid HIV tests and whether such testing changes behavior or improves public health. We don't know whether diabetic people who closely monitor their glucose levels live any longer than those who don't. We don't know whether women who test themselves for urinary-tract infections have better outcomes.

And now, as at-home genetic tests hit the market, we have little idea how people will use or misuse the complex information these products offer. Before other groundbreaking tests like the pregnancy kit and the rapid HIV detection test became available to consumers, they faced a lengthy FDA approval process and push-back from the medical industry. This may explain why many of the consumer-genomics companies insist that they're not offering medical services. For instance, 23andMe's consent form states that what the company offers "is not a test or kit designed to diagnose disease or medical conditions, and it is not intended to be medical advice."

According to Dr. Muin Khoury, director of the National Office of Public Health Genomics at the Centers for Disease Control and Prevention in Atlanta, the information provided by DTC companies is mostly useless—and potentially harmful. Khoury is most concerned about tests that offer advice on health-related issues, such as screening and risk assessment that may lead to clinical interventions. "These tests are not ready for prime time—that's the bottom line," he says. "I've said this many times and in many articles in the past few years. The currently available tests are not predictive enough to be useful for screening."

Although skeptical, he concedes that the tests can also be helpful—sometimes. Khoury tells the story of a man he knows who took such a test and learned that he had an increased risk of prostate cancer. On the surface, this particular case doesn't seem to be that significant or newsworthy, but it triggered a wave of publicity because the man, Jeffrey Gulcher, happens to be the chief science officer for deCODE Genetics, one of the DTC companies. Spontaneously, one day Gulcher spat into a test tube, paid his $850 and sent the sample to his company's lab for analysis. Gulcher was only forty-eight, and men aren't usually in jeopardy for prostate cancer until later in life. He was also unaware of any history of prostate cancer in his family. But several weeks later, when the test results were returned, Gulcher was shocked to learn that he had a genetic variant that literally doubled his lifetime risk of contracting prostate cancer— from the normal 15% to 30%. To be clear, this test didn't say he had prostate cancer or would get it—only that based on current data, he was more likely to develop cancer than the average man his age.

And even though he was well aware of the caveats, Gulcher panicked and went to his physician, who did a blood test. The physician then referred Gulcher to a urologist for an exploratory biopsy—and just in time. His prostate gland was riddled with cancer, which seemed poised to begin spreading. Gulcher scheduled a prostatectomy, utterly convinced that DTC genetic testing had actually saved his life. Was he right? Perhaps.

Khoury won't say that Gulcher was wrong—only that the situation is not so cut and dried and doesn't really prove a lot. He points out that men can live long lives with prostate cancer and die from other causes. And removing the prostate has risks, including impotence. Gulcher could have maintained his health and life without taking action. So what's a doctor to do? Order surgery for all patients with gene profiles indicating high risk of prostate cancer? The cost would be astronomical, especially considering the fact that the utility of these tests has not been proven.

Gulcher, for example, learned that he had a higher-than-average chance of contracting prostate cancer—not that he was going to get prostate cancer. In truth, research shows that two thirds of men whose lifetime risk for prostate cancer is double the average—like Gulcher's—will not contract prostate cancer or, if they do, it will occur much later in life and present itself in such a benign form that treatment will be unnecessary. That said, comfort with risk is highly individual, and each consumer or patient has to decide what amount of risk is going to motivate him to act——for Gulcher, 30% was enough—and then determine the action he might take.

Prostate cancer is especially confusing, these days, because of the controversy surrounding PSA tests; in October 2011, the US Preventive Services Task Force recommended that otherwise healthy men not be screened regularly, due to a lack of proof that such screening actually saves lives. And yet, prostate cancer casts a dark shadow over all middle-aged men. Screening may not be effective on a society-wide level—but what if you, as an individual, could save your life by being cautious, as Gulcher believes he did?

Michael Saks would soon face a similar conundrum in the process of learning more about his genetic heritage. Saks, however, feared an even more threatening and insidious type of cancer.

CHAPTER 9:
BIOMARKER BAKE-OFF

A way to distinguish between normal cells and cancer cells in the body is to imagine two brothers. They could be twins, they look so much alike—except that one brother is a homebody and the other is a migrant traveler. The homebody brother is the normal cell; like the mortals they inhabit, these cells grow for a while, slow down when they mature, live a quiet and largely productive life and eventually die. They remain close to home from beginning to end.

In contrast, the cancer cell may travel incessantly, migrating throughout the body. As it travels, the cancer cell becomes evil—poisonous—and begins to take on different recognizable and threatening characteristics. What's even more depressing and frightening is the fact that unlike normal cells, cancer cells become nearly immortal; they will survive as long as there are nutrients to sustain them—and the longer they survive the more they divide, or metastasize. The way in which they divide is controlled by one certain type of gene—a "checkpoint gene"—which may be termed the universal arbitrator, or mechanism, for all cell division in virtually all organisms from mere fungi to human beings.

The scientist who received much of the credit for discovering and isolating this mechanism is Leland (Lee) H. Hartwell, who, in 2001, was presented with the Nobel Prize in Physiology of Medicine for his co-discovery (with Tim Hunt and Sir Paul M. Nurse) of checkpoint genes—vital information for scientists and physicians seeking to understand the mechanisms of cancer and the way we think about life itself. Like the friar Gregor Mendel, who conducted breeding experiments with peas from his garden, Hartwell performed his experiments using a common and seemingly unlikely organism, which, like Mendel's peas, was nevertheless complex enough to relate to human development. Hartwell chose yeast, a single-celled fungus which bakers use to make bread dough rise and brewers and winemakers use to ferment their products.

At the time he received the Nobel Prize, Hartwell was president and director of the Fred Hutchinson Cancer Research Center in Seattle, Washington. Both accomplishments—the Nobel and his appointment as leader of "The Hutch," generally acknowledged as one of the world's premier basic cancer research institutions—could be considered crowning achievements in his very prestigious and accomplished life. His was a rags-to-riches American story: Hartwell, from humble beginnings, was the first person in his family to go to college.

Growing up in southern California, Lee Hartwell's passions included auto mechanics and butterflies—quite a combination. If the teenage Hartwell—slender, wiry and athletic—could not be found tinkering with an engine under the hood of an old jalopy in a grimy garage, he'd be in a meadow somewhere, collecting bugs, butterflies, snakes and spiders. He was also drawn to books, although as a pragmatist, he often did not believe exactly what he read, a lesson he learned by accepting the notion presented in one high school biology textbook which observed that lizards lacked teeth. One day, he snared a very large lizard and watched in surprise and then pain as the lizard opened his mouth and sank its teeth deep into his thumb. But Hartwell was undeterred, becoming increasingly intrigued with the secrets of science. Even as a young teenager he wanted to understand it all on a fundamental level. "I used to get annoyed at my father, a neon-sign man," he remembers, "because he would not explain to me how neon signs work. I only realized later that I wanted to know about electricity and atomic emissions, topics that he knew nothing about."

After high school, Hartwell started taking classes at Glendale Junior College and eventually did well enough to receive a scholarship to California Institute of Technology, where he did his undergraduate work. In 1964 he earned a PhD from the Massachusetts Institute of Technology; then he did postdoctoral work at the Salk Institute for Biological Studies from 1964 through 1965, and joined the University of Washington faculty in 1968. In 1996 he joined the faculty of Seattle's Fred Hutchinson Cancer Research Center and in 1997 became its president and director. From the teenage boy puzzling over the secrets of neon to the Nobel Laureate unraveling the secrets of life itself, Lee Hartwell has never for an instant lost his fascination with science, hungering to understand its fundamentals, which he has called "magical."

* * *

The idea that science is spiritual (as Francis Collins might contend) or "magical" (as Hartwell puts it) could be debated. But there is certainly an abundance of mystery in scientific research—and, even more than mystery, an onslaught of hard work, persistence, faith, hope, dedication and luck. The history of cancer over the centuries is full of theories to which scientists have devoted entire careers only to end up at a dead end. But in science, at least, a dead end often leads to a new beginning.

This is a major reason why I admire scientists so much, and why we must continue to fuel their passion—research—because they never give up in their quest for knowledge that will lead to vital breakthroughs in understanding. What I appreciate even more is that there's rarely an end point to their obsession. Hartwell is a poster child for this obsessive drive. Leland Hartwell's work with checkpoint genes did shed light on a key aspect of cancer, but cancer continues to be the second-leading cause of death in Americans. And so Hartwell and thousands of his colleagues continue working in laboratories and clinics and seeking new answers, which lead to more questions, a process never ending.

We can trace the search for a cure or at least a better understanding of cancer a long way back—beginning perhaps with Claudius Galen, a Greek physician and a writer who settled in Rome in the second century AD Like the ancient Greek physician Hippocrates, Galen was convinced that four bodily fluids (or "humors") determined the state of health of an individual—and that disease and a dark mood were caused by an imbalance of these fluids.

Treating the patient back then began with an assessment of the four fluids. A "blood" person was optimistic and passionate, while a person with lots of "phlegm" was just the opposite—dull and sluggish. People with too much "yellow bile" had terrible tempers, while "black bile" caused melancholy and depression. Black bile was the most dreaded of the fluids because it was also, according Hippocrates, the primary cause of cancer.

In a way, you can make a comparison between ancient medicine, with its four humors, and modern medicine, which is increasingly based around the four building blocks of DNA. We have made progress, to be sure, but we are still, in many ways, completely ignorant. We have made significant advances in keeping patients alive, and we have gathered a mountain of information—but we haven't cured cancer. Not by a long shot.

Galen was a prolific writer who wrote so extensively and convincingly about Hippocrates's cancer/black bile connection that these ideas about cancer were accepted for well over 1,000 years—all the way through the Middle Ages. It was not until the middle of the sixteenth century, in fact, when a Belgian student, Andreas Vesalius, arrived in Paris to study to be a surgeon, that doctors' understanding of cancer began to change. Vesalius had been nearly obsessed by Galen's ideas and his writings since childhood. Medicine, like art and sports, can inspire young people, one disciple after another, in that way. When he arrived to study at the University of Paris, however, Vesalius discovered that surgery was taught by trial and error. It involved mostly guesswork, and little precision. Surgeons sliced their way through cadavers without any clear idea of where they were going or what they might find in the body. They taught themselves—some, as you might imagine, more successfully than others.

There were only a few general anatomical sketches of the body available at that time and, Vesalius discovered, many of those were inaccurate. This inspired Vesalius to begin a lifelong quest to produce precise maps of every part of the human anatomy. His method of study was an obsession and somewhat of a scandal, as well, since the only way to do his work was to forage through graveyards and walk the streets and highways secretly seeking legs, arms and bones—any body part was a treasure. The more drawings and sketches he made, the more demand there was for him to do more—and to focus on organs, nerves and blood vessels.

There was a method to his madness, however—a mission. All the while, Vesalius was seeking evidence of the fluids that Galen had described—and to a certain extent, he was successful. Vesalius found yellow bile in the liver, blood in arteries and veins, and pale and watery phlegm-like fluid in the lymphatic system. But, alas, he could find no black bile in the entire body, wherever he looked—and therefore no cause or root of cancer. This had been the most significant of Galen's claims—the most memorable and vivid—and Andreas Vesalius disproved it.

The irony was clear. He had devoted his life to anatomy in order to prove that Galen was right and that black bile caused cancer, but in the end he demonstrated the exact opposite. This was not a bad thing, of course; in the long quest to understand cancer, this represented significant progress.

Subsequently, many other ways to see the inside of the patient and begin to figure out how the vast and complicated human mechanism works (or doesn't work) have been developed: X-rays; microscopes that can help scientists scrutinize cancer cells and determine their pathology; Magnetic Resonance Imaging (MRI); and, most recently, molecular diagnostics. And today scientists are talking about protein biomarkers.

Remember that proteins do most of the work in cells and are essential to the structure, function and regulation of the body's tissues and organs. Proteins can recognize and frequently protect the body from foreign or dangerous molecules.

Biomarkers are simply protein molecules that can be found in the blood, other body fluids and tissues, and analyzed for presence of disease, infection or environmental exposure.

In simple terms, biomarkers are like breadcrumbs, microscopic signals or indications that can be used to measure a biological process—which means, essentially, something happening in the body during the development of a disease or a response to a medicine. In oncology, biomarkers can determine prognosis, how patients may respond to certain medications, how aggressively a patient needs to be treated, how rapidly the disease is likely to progress and even how long a patient might live. In chronic lymphocytic leukemia, the most common adult leukemia, for example, about half of patients have a mutation affecting the immunoglobulin gene, and these patients tend to live longer than patients lacking the mutation—and the recognition of the gene, our ability to see and analyze it, comes through biomarkers.

Another example, according to the American Society of Clinical Oncology: routinely testing people with colon cancer for mutations of one very active gene (the *KRAS* oncogene) would save approximately $600 million annually and spare patients futile, painful and sometimes toxic treatments.

The more we see the inner workings of the body, the more we understand how the body works—and how and when it doesn't work—and how scientists and physicians can intervene. I think we can say that the search for a cure for cancer has been going on since Hippocrates; in essence, modern civilization has been one long crusade to examine, in increasing depth and detail, the way in which the human body functions. In many ways, biomarkers mean to medicine today what Vesalius's anatomical maps meant to physicians in the early days of the Renaissance; both represent the state of the art in their time.

Why are biomarkers better than genes to study? Hartwell gives many reasons. DNA reveals only hereditary predispositions to disease, whereas proteins can determine when disease strikes and how thoroughly it has progressed in an individual. Mathematically, one gene can produce a family of many variant proteins, adding to the amount of the diagnostic information available. Proteins are less invasive and expensive to procure, for they can be isolated in the bloodstream, whereas DNA is mostly obtained by biopsy of the diseased tissue. This issue of invasiveness is quite important; a biopsy is a surgical procedure and every procedure, no matter how routine, contains a measure of danger. Heart transplant recipients, for example, often need multiple biopsies in any given year to monitor for organ rejection. Sometimes these are taken as often as once a week, especially early on, causing suffering and pain, not to mention expense, in regular intervals. A blood test has now been developed (AlloMap) to replace the necessity of biopsy in some patients. Someday soon, perhaps, there will be biomarkers to detect prostate cancer, as Lawrence Brody has suggested, and biomarkers to take the place of an ubiquitous and invasive procedure—colonoscopy.

Biomarkers will be especially valuable in diagnostic areas, which is exactly where Hartwell wants to go—into prevention rather than therapeutics. The reality is that treatment drugs are more valuable than diagnostics to medical centers and pharmaceutical companies, not to mention to scientists seeking research support. The bottom line is that it's more profitable to treat (and hope to cure) a disease, than to anticipate or prevent it. This is a reality that annoys and motivates Hartwell and may well be a motivation for the shift in his career and his move to Arizona.

I first witnessed Hartwell in action in March 2010 at the Biltmore Hotel in Phoenix, at a conference sponsored by the American Association of the Advancement of Science (AAAS): Personalized Medicine in the Clinic: Policy, Legal and Ethical Implications. Hartwell was keynote speaker; the title of his talk was The Promise and Progress of Personalized Medicine.

Considering his position as the Virginia G. Piper chair in personalized medicine and chief scientist at ASU's Center for Sustainable Health, I hunkered down and waited for what I expected to be a glowing outline of the future of personalized medicine.

The Virginia G. Piper Charitable Trust, incidentally, the foundation for which Dr. Lee Hartwell's chair had been named, has many interests, but healthcare and medical research in the Maricopa County area in Arizona has been a primary focus. Lee Hartwell, while still directing the Fred Hutchinson Cancer Research Center in Seattle, Washington, served as an adviser to Piper Trust. In September 2007, the trust announced an award of $10 million to ASU and $20 million to the Translational Genomics Research Institute (TGen) to support the Partnership of Personalized Medicine. Subsequently the Trust has awarded additional funds to support the establishment of ASU's Center for Sustainable Health and Lee Hartwell as its Virginia G. Piper chair and chief scientist of personalized medicine. A second Piper chair in personalized medicine was established for Dr. Joshua LaBaer, who was recruited to ASU's Biodesign Institute. LaBaer was director of the Harvard Institute of Proteomics.

I expected Hartwell's keynote address to report plenty of progress and a tidal wave of promise. But it wasn't that at all, surprisingly. Hartwell was quite cautionary. Many of the attendees I talked with at the conference—more than 200 nurses, physicians, hospital administrators and pharmaceutical company executives attended—were similarly surprised by the talk, and in some ways relieved that they were not being asked to learn or adopt something that could not be applied to their industry and practice for at least another decade, or longer in some cases.

Hartwell put that into perspective. I was especially struck by the metaphor he used to describe the future of personalized medicine: he began his talk by comparing the personalized medicine movement to a train that had just left the train station. But, he cautioned, "It is a very slow train with a very long way to go, and we will need to do some track switches along the way before we arrive at our destination."

At another conference the following year, also at the Biltmore, Hartwell repeated the same train metaphor. In fact, the brochure for the conference, the Forum for Sustainable Health, was designed as a bullet train leaving a station. And at that forum, Hartwell had another metaphor: a relay race— four groups united with the challenge of changing the healthcare system and of not losing momentum as they achieve their goals and hand off the baton to one another. This is part of Hartwell's mission—and not a particularly likely prospect for the moment. But the four groups—government officials, the pharmaceutical industry, the computer industry, and physicians and academic scientists—were all represented at the forum, and just bringing all of those groups together for an "off-the-record" conversation was in itself quite an achievement.

In some ways an idealist, Hartwell is quite pragmatic and realistic in his refusal to buy into the hype of genomics. He acknowledges the fact that sequencing the genome was a monumental feat, which has opened up many doors and advanced science in many important ways. Unlike many of his colleagues, however, who predict that affordable genomic sequencing will usher in imminent breakthroughs, Hartwell adamantly rejects this thesis: "That's completely wrong." Sequencing of the genome in every person, Hartwell believes, will provide some—*some*—valuable information about the ways in which cancers and other diseases differ and how to treat them, which can be vital; but he insists that the research is not as useful as it is cracked up to be. In his view, if the HGP proved anything, it showed how massive amounts of information can cause many more questions and problems than answers and breakthroughs. Hartwell says that research into genetics will continue and occasionally provide useful medical information, but it is time that we forge ahead beyond the genes. He builds a strong case, in fact, in both scientific and social action directions.

Hartwell is relaxed, easygoing and casual, and he has a soft, rather high-pitched style of speaking that makes people lean forward and pay more attention. He is self-effacing and has an engaging wit.

On the night of his Nobel acceptance, Hartwell was handsome and natty in formal attire, but most often he is seen wearing blue jeans or khakis and a tieless white shirt—sometimes with a blue blazer. His clothes often seem too big for him, as if he were shrinking. A road biker who commutes to work on two wheels, Hartwell at seventy is slender and fit with wavy silver hair and an easy smile, but he is clearly a man who knows what he knows.

Hartwell is disturbed by the fact that most of the progress being made in science has had a minimal benefit on medicine and the healthcare system, and he wants to change that reality. Instead of using our assets to prevent disease, the entire healthcare system is based upon late-stage interventions—what to do after patients like Michael Saks's mother are diagnosed with pancreatic cancer. In other words, after the damage is done. We've expended trillions of dollars on research and treatment in the last stage of life, the final year—by 2015, according to the Partnership of Personalized Medicine, about one fifth of the United States domestic product will be devoted to healthcare and four fifths of that amount to late-stage treatment.

Hartwell believes that biomarkers could be the key to changing the way medicine is practiced. And yet, as certain as Hartwell is about the importance of biomarkers, he also admits that we have a long way to go to be able to use them in medicine across the board. We are only in the very beginning stages of the protein biomarker era, specifically, or molecular diagnostics, generally. Hartwell's colleague, George Poste, who founded the ASU Biodesign Institute, recently wrote an article in *Nature*, pointing out that since the introduction of technologies such as proteomics and DNA microarrays, more than 150,000 papers have been published, documenting thousands of biomarkers, but fewer than one hundred have been validated for clinical practice. As in much of personalized medicine, we are faced with a fundamental challenge: basic raw data that we don't know what to do with or how to narrow down and define. Or, to put it another way: information without application.

"If you study the literature," says Hartwell, "you will find thousands of reports of people from research laboratories who did a study of a group of patients and found molecules that are likely to be a good biomarker. But then the studies die. Nobody takes them any further—and somebody has to," says Hartwell. "It is such a waste of effort otherwise."

As an example, Hartwell isolates colon cancer. "With cancer, the name of the game is 'detect it early,' and we can do that 70% of the time with colonoscopy. But that is a couple of thousand dollars a shot. Pretty expensive, pretty invasive; so most people don't do it. So what you need is a much simpler blood test or some kind of test with a stool that reveals the presence of cancer." Hartwell says that such a test will be coming fairly soon, but laments that it has been slow in coming—it might have happened a while ago.

Hartwell admits that at this time scientists haven't the slightest idea how many biomarkers exist within the human body or where they can be found. Every disease may have a dozen biomarker signals—and perhaps more. As Poste noted, every day researchers around the world turn up new biomarkers, connected in one tangential way or another to many diseases and mutations.

At the AAAS meeting, Hartwell suggested a biomarker "bake-off"—in essence, to take a particular disease, examine all of the literature related to the hundreds and perhaps thousands of studies and discoveries of biomarkers around that disease, develop a procedure to identify the most informative and promising studies and test the most promising of the reported biomarkers around that set. Then scientists can move forward either by conducting research on their own or by attempting to involve commercial partners, such as pharmaceutical companies. This is no easy feat, however, since genes and proteins (and therefore biomarkers) can change, somewhat arbitrarily. It seems that a person's experience, including where they live and what they eat, can generate chemicals that attach to the genes and cause the change. As I have said, unraveling the mystery of the human body seems to be a never-ending, and increasingly complicated, endeavor—and Hartwell remains in the heat of it.

Hunting, cataloguing and developing biomarkers is only part of Hartwell's plan, however. He envisions a national biosignatures laboratory, where protein biomarkers identified in intensive comparative evidence-based studies in medical centers can be recorded and catalogued. What Hartwell means by biosignatures is a more panoramic collection of indicators that lead to disease. This would include not only the broad scope of molecular diagnostics, but also medical history and information relating to the patient's behavior—in short, everything you ever needed to know about a patient, that was asked or that you forgot to ask.

Hartwell distinguishes between a biosignatures laboratory and a biobank. Some scientists and government administrators are campaigning for a US biobank, which would house and preserve a massive collection of blood and tissue samples of every American. A number of countries are far ahead of the United States in this endeavor, with Iceland leading the way, primarily because its population is so homogeneous, and so small. England's biobank has more than 500,000 registered. But how tissue and other material is collected and subsequently stored is not regulated or standardized, so Hartwell and others question how useful those samples will be for scientific research and medical diagnostics.

Efforts like Hartwell's national biosignatures laboratory, however, are actually underway in this country; the idea is not as pie-in-the-sky as it sounds. These days, patients at Harvard's Brigham and Women's Hospital, for example, are asked if they want to voluntarily contribute a blood sample for genetic testing. The hospital started this effort with great moderation—recruiting fewer than 1,000 patients, but their goal is to have a data bank with samples from more than 100,000 patients, data all devoted to understanding how genes influence health. Brigham epidemiologists intend to link this information to each patient's electronic medical record and then follow and monitor each patient over a long period of time, adding information, when available, about lifestyle and environment.

A sister institution in Boston, Children's Hospital, has initiated a similar effort. Children's Hospital of Philadelphia has been building a similar database and has already enlisted a population of more than 50,000 children—with a goal of doubling the size. All of this information, by the way, will be used only for research, and will not be available to patients or their families—a decision that is certain to cause significant legal difficulties and objections down the line.

Despite the obstacles, this is the kind of collection Hartwell envisions. He is particularly concerned with adding environmental influences. For although genetics are significant, Hartwell stresses the incredible divergences caused by environment: "The incidence of lung cancer in New Orleans is 110 cases per 100,000 population annually while the incidence in lung cancer in China per 100,000 population annually is 6." A long-range study of native Japanese who migrated to Hawaii demonstrated that it's "not the people who carry the cancer, but where they reside."

According to epigeneticist Michael Skinner of Washington State University, almost every region in the world has different disease frequencies. In Japan, there is a very high rate of stomach disease and a very low rate of prostate disease. If you take someone early in life and transfer them from Japan to the United States, they will more likely have prostate troubles and are less likely to fall victim to stomach diseases. Food also enters into the roots of genetic heritage. Foods eaten in Western Europe, for instance, are quite different from foods eaten in China, Korea and Japan—factors that eventually influence genetic make-up.

And even on a genetic level, some populations are more vulnerable to certain mutations than others, for reasons that are not yet clear. Scientists don't know why Europeans who inherit two copies (one from each side of the family) of *APOE-ε4*, the "Alzheimer's Gene," are fifteen times more likely to develop Alzheimer's disease than Hispanics and African-Americans who have inherited the gene from both sides. Doctors are still studying why it seems Japanese with the same two-copy inheritance are even less likely to develop Alzheimer's than Hispanics and African-Americans.

Crohn's, an inflammatory bowel disease, presents a similar quandary—with a difference. Three disease-causing variants have been associated with Crohn's disease in Europeans, but none of these variants have yet been discovered in Chinese, Korean or Japanese populations. Perhaps this too has something to do with intermarriage—or the lack thereof in frequency between Asians and Europeans. But it might also have something to do with food or the air they breathe—or even their leisure activities, like smoking and drinking.

But the best predictive factor to disease? Says Hartwell, the oldest and most tried-and-true factor: family history.

Steve Murphy could have told him that—although Murphy probably doesn't want hear to Hartwell's prediction regarding private-practice physicians.

Hartwell thinks that the private-practice physician will someday be replaced by a few minor drugstore diagnostics. "I think someday you'll go into a drugstore, and, like you take your blood pressure today, there will be someday be a little machine," he says. "Put in your money and out pops a computer printout that says you better go see your kidney doctor—or whoever. Similar scenarios go in different directions. There's the patient, for example, who picks up a hand-held device and, with a slight pinprick, siphons off a droplet of blood and sends it off to a distant supercomputer for an analysis of anywhere from 1,000 to 5,000 different aspects. The information goes to the patient's personal physician who, if noting something untoward, may send advice and direction. This scenario assumes the existence of the personal physician, but he or she probably won't be the same person we know as our family doctor today.

"I think we will soon eliminate the general practitioner because they're really crude diagnosticians," says Hartwell. "They look at your temperature and your heartbeat and they try to predict what's going on and where does it hurt. You won't need that. You'll go directly from the drugstore to the specialist."

This will not be particularly good news to Steve Murphy, although by the time this happens, if it ever happens, chances are Murphy will be in a rocking chair and his children will be in practice. And perhaps they will call themselves biomedical engineers or biosignature analysts. "Medical doctor" may no longer seem quite complete enough.

CHAPTER 10:
THE CONTEXT
OF VULNERABILITY

The words "tumor" and "malignant" may be two of the most awful and frightening words a person can ever hear. Those words most often mean cancer, and cancer means pain and suffering and, all too often, death. In Galen's day, we knew very little about tumors, although he did recognize them and write about them, in *De tumoribus praeter naturam*. Later, when Vesalius began capturing every tiny detail of the human body, he concentrated on the normal body rather than the abnormal. And a tumor is nothing if not abnormal; because it multiplies and divides rather indiscriminately, a tumor, whether benign or malignant, is larger than all of the cells around it. You recognize a tumor because it stands out; it is different by its size and shape. (By color, at least, it is usually neutral, mostly what you'd expect: fatty tissue and rivulets of blood.)

More than two centuries after Vesalius, the Scottish physician Matthew Baillie wrote and illustrated a book for surgeons that was the antithesis of Vesalius's study of the normal body. *The Morbid Anatomy of Some of the Most Important Parts of the Human Body* was a catalogue of the body in its abnormal, or diseased, state. Baillie categorized tumors, albeit quite generally. Tumors of the lung stood out, "large as an orange," he said, while tumors in the stomach took on a "fungous" appearance, meaning that they were somewhat spongy.

In 2008, Sue, a victim of breast cancer, wrote in her blog, *Sue's Escape from Cancerland*: "If someone had asked a year ago, what color the inside of a tumor was, I would have guessed red and gray. When they did the biopsy, I asked to see the tissue specimens: five quarter- to half-inch strings of vermicelli (Italian for little worms) with little streakings of blood. They didn't look evil to me, just strings of fat. The entire mass was white inside as the pathology report stated."

But despite how innocent they looked, the tumors—her tumors—were "evil," Sue wrote. And that assessment seems to me to be the best way to describe a tumor. When I think of a tumor I do not envision it first under a microscope; I think of the devil incarnate—red faced, with menacing horns and fire in his eyes. Perhaps it was a similar belief—that the tumor was too big and evil and ugly to be inside a person—that drove early surgeons to do everything in their power to cut the tumor out, to exorcise the demon from the body. Thus, for a long time, surgeons were the physicians of record for cancer.

The beginning to middle of the nineteenth century was a crucial period in the history of surgery, as surgeons learned to perform effective transfusions, which kept patients from excessive blood loss; developed more effective anesthesia; and learned how to combat infection. In 1882, William Stewart Halsted performed the first successful radical breast mastectomy, which remains a frightening chapter in the history of breast cancer surgery. He removed entire shoulders and chests, literally, to rid the body of the dreaded (but no longer completely invincible) malignant tumor that could metastasize throughout the body.

The lumpectomy—surgery in which only the tumor and the surrounding tissue is removed—did not become an established procedure in breast cancer until the early 1980s. The idea of chemotherapy, the notion that you could actually destroy the tumor inside of the body with powerful poisonous fluids and compounds, was not really proven to be effective until the late 1950s and1960s. Official recognition of medical oncology as a new subspecialty of internal medicine took place in 1972, and gradually surgeons have faded from the forefront of the cancer picture.

Even in the best of modern times, however, chemotherapy is often ineffective—and there are many times when chemotherapy itself is also a problem, nearly as damaging and dangerous as the tumor itself. And no wonder. The first chemotherapy treatments were made from poisonous cloth dyes in the nineteenth century. And early in the twentieth century, scientists were experimenting with nitrogen mustard as a chemotherapy agent; it became better known as mustard gas on the front lines in France and Germany in World War I. Today, of course, there are much more sophisticated compounds to treat tumors, but we all know from friends and family, and perhaps from personal experience, that even the mildest chemotherapy detonates inside the body, causing massive trauma—and then, despite the pain, the weakness, the exhaustion and hair loss it causes, sometimes it doesn't work.

But notice the progression: from black bile to biomarkers, from radical mastectomy to targeted compounds, we continue to study the body and the tumor ever more closely, digging increasingly deeper not only to visualize the cancers that threaten and kill hundreds of thousands of Americans every year but also to learn how to defeat it without the devastation of surgery. This is where personalized medicine is taking us, where it has already taken us—to a point in time when we are beginning to understand the enemy, the tumor, and to demonstrate that it is not invincible.

And tumors are not invincible; that's worth repeating. They have weak points that can sometimes be targeted and destroyed or incapacitated. Remember the Greek warrior Achilles, who was seemingly invincible during the Trojan War, but eventually died because of a small wound in his heel? Some tumors, scientists have discovered, and maybe all tumors, have a weak point, an Achilles heel. If you can find this weak point and target it with a medication tailored to that tumor, you can knock the tumor out—without knocking the patient out. Oncologists often point out that the "P" word "personalized" should be replaced by another, more accurate "P" word—"precision." For this is what is supposed to be happening in personalized medicine—finding the point of vulnerability, then tailoring a medication that will be effective and sending it like a missile to the target. This is the idea that Michael Saks was drawn to when he first heard the lecturer from the Biodesign Institute describe the future of medicine, though Saks has since come to realize—and doctors and researchers throughout the United States would admit it—we've still got a long way to go.

But the process is rapidly moving ahead at places like TGen, the Translational Genomics Research Institute, in Scottsdale, Arizona. TGen was founded in 2002; the president and research director, Dr. Jeffrey Trent, was formerly the scientific director of the National Human Genomics Research Institute. But the leading clinical figure at TGen, one of its cofounders, is oncologist Daniel D. Von Hoff, who is physician-in-chief and distinguished professor there. In addition, Von Hoff is the chief scientific officer for the Scottsdale Healthcare Research Institute, as well as a clinical professor of medicine at the University of Arizona and chief scientific officer for US Oncology.

Von Hoff arrived in Phoenix around the same time as Hartwell began directing the Hutch. He had been a clinician at the University of Texas Health Science Center at San Antonio, and his primary goal and mission was, then and now, to develop therapeutic agents to diagnose and cure pancreatic cancer. Von Hoff and TGen have been developing drugs for cancers other than pancreatic cancer, as well. At a research facility like TGen, you find an agent—a drug—and you break it down into microscopic parts, and test it against all sorts of tumors, alone and in combination with other agents, hoping to find a way in which it might, somehow, be effective.

Von Hoff and Hartwell are approximately the same age and they are certainly on the same wavelength; their missions in life are in lockstep, but their personalities and the organizations they represent are very different in many ways. Hartwell's Center for Sustainable Health is more like a think tank filled with what some people might describe as overly ambitious expectations of changing the healthcare system, putting prevention in front of procedures.

In contrast, the clinical aspect of TGen, based at the Scottsdale Medical Center, is the grittiest and most in-the-trenches kind of work. The patients who come to be treated by Dr. Von Hoff are offering themselves as guinea pigs, for many of the therapies Von Hoff and TGen provide are experimental drugs in the first phase of clinical trials or experimentation.

In many ways having a personalized medicine or genomics think tank and a last-resort, in-the-trenches cancer facility—and having very little middle ground (a major medical center, for example)—is very "Arizona." The world's vision of Arizona is as a state somewhat out of control with gun-wielding crazies running amok, beginning with Sheriff Joe Arpaio, famous for his tent city concentration camp of prisoners in Maricopa County. Then alongside Sheriff Joe there's the wealthy retiree population and hundreds of golf courses in every direction, within tee shots of one another. And plenty of students—Arizona State University possesses the largest student body in a university in the United States, nearly 80,000 undergraduate and graduate students. But the cowboy culture is pervasive. I am speaking here as an insider—although I have only been around for a couple of years as a member of a science policy think tank, the Consortium of Science Policy & Outcomes.

TGen, incidentally, has been supported by the state of Arizona and many foundations, including the Virginia G. Piper Charitable Trust and the Flinn Foundation, which, like Piper, has also been active in supporting and promoting the advancement of the biosciences in Arizona. The existence of TGen has also contributed a great deal to the region's economy. A report recently released by Tripp Umbach, a national leader in economic forecasting, estimated that TGen provides Arizona with a total annual economic impact of $137.7 million. It is an interesting development in an area which, until very recently, did not have a medical school or the complement of faculty, residents, students and patients that ordinarily are a part of such an institution.

I can't compare Hartwell or Von Hoff to Sheriff Joe, but in some respects Von Hoff and Hartwell are also cowboys, roaming the biomedical frontier—one on a very high plane as the thinker, Hartwell, and the other low in the desert (the doer)—looking for answers to problems that no one else in the nation can solve. And they are both obsessed and driven—just like Steve Murphy.

At TGen and the Scottsdale Healthcare Research Institute and the Virginia G. Piper Cancer Center, where he does his clinical work, Von Hoff focuses much of his attention on patients involved in Phase I drug trials—when patients are in the most trouble and the closest to death.

According to the FDA, Phase I is when scientists begin looking into the value or the activity of a drug—the initial phase that determines the rate at which the drug is metabolized, its potential toxicity and any early evidence of effectiveness. The number of subjects in a Phase I trial typically ranges from twenty to eighty. If Phase I studies don't reveal unacceptable toxicity, Phase II studies begin. While the emphasis in Phase I is on safety, the emphasis in Phase II is on effectiveness. Typically, the number of subjects in Phase II studies ranges from 100 to about 300. Then, if evidence of effectiveness is shown in Phase II, Phase III studies begin. These studies gather more information about safety and effectiveness, studying different populations and different dosages and using the drug in combination with other drugs. The number of subjects usually ranges from 1,000 to about 3,000 people.

The FDA states that "Phase I studies are usually conducted in healthy volunteers." But this is kind of tricky, because the healthiest volunteers are generally not particularly interested in doing guinea pig duty on substances about which they and their physicians know very little—not even the extent of their toxicity. Because of its bench-to-bedside orientation, however, TGen is often in the process of conducting Phase I trials that, because of the drugs' inherent experimental nature, will most often be tried on patients who have gone through all of the more tried-and-true therapies without much success. Most folks who arrive at Von Hoff's doorstep—TGen will accept most any patient, as long as they are comparatively healthy—are circling the drain. If something doesn't happen soon—perhaps they will rally, or the drug that Von Hoff tries on them will work temporarily—the truth of the matter is that most of the patients who come to TGen for help have less than three months to live.

Von Hoff is stocky and broad shouldered, anchored to the ground like a fireplug; balding, with bushy silver brows that jiggle in a frenzied state when he tells a story; and he has the pasty complexion of a man who spends too much time indoors in a laboratory or clinic. A total opposite of Hartwell in looks and demeanor, Von Hoff is intense, outgoing and energetic—excessively so. When he tells a story, which he does quite frequently, he becomes so involved he acts many of the parts out. I once saw him on national TV in a CBS *Stand Up to Cancer* special hosted by Katie Couric. At the end of the show, the participants—patients, doctors, nurses, family members—gathered onstage for what can only be described as a cheering session or pep rally, like on a football field, but for curing cancer. Many of the physicians and older folks stood by and fidgeted or went through the cheering motions when the signal was given and the marching band music was being played, but Von Hoff became as crazed as the teenagers, screaming and cheering for their mutual dreams for the future.

In many ways the pep rally seemed overly optimistic. Yes, cancer researchers are making new discoveries every day, but for many patients, a diagnosis of cancer is still a death sentence. Personally, I have had three friends diagnosed with pancreatic cancer over the past two years. One of them is already dead. The other two have unoptimistic prognoses. I asked Von Hoff if he really believed that pancreatic cancer could be cured in his lifetime, given the dismal statistics and the constant setbacks. "I don't intend to retire until it happens," he told me.

Von Hoff explains how to isolate the tumor's Achilles heel, a process he calls identifying the "contexts of vulnerability." There are the genetic, the environmental and the molecular contexts of vulnerability—which are sometimes three totally separate avenues to probe. The process begins with listening to the patient and taking a good history, which is pretty much what any other physician would say, although according to his staff, Von Hoff takes this very seriously—devoting hours to new patients in order to get their story straight and to make certain they are comfortable. He will sometimes stand in front of a whiteboard with a Magic Marker and teach his patients what they need to know about their tumors and the substances they will be ingesting.

But first, he listens: if a patient has an Ashkenazi Jewish background, for example, *BRCA1* and *BRCA2* are serious and obvious considerations. The genetic underpinnings can tell the physician what the patient is susceptible to and, to a certain extent, how to treat it. For example, one strain of lung cancer is more common in nonsmoking Asian women than in any other population. "So an Asian woman walks into my office and says, 'I got lung cancer and I never smoked in my life,' I'm immediately thinking epidermal growth factor receptor mutation," Von Hoff says. "Very common and easy to take care of. You can give her a drug that hits that mutation, 80% of the time shrink the tumor, no side effects. It's amazing. So this particular drug matches this particular type of tumor—that's targeting the tumor's Achilles heel.

"But if a Camel-smoking man comes in, a guy who smoked all his life, or even an American guy who has been smoke free, but has lung cancer, I've got nothing for him. Why? Well, it is a different mutation than the one the Asian woman has." Can the Camel smoking man ever have that mutation? "Sometimes they do—about 2% of the time. It's 80% for her but 2% for him. Not particularly good odds."

When I first met him, Von Hoff immediately threw two terms into the personalized medicine mix that had nothing to do with science or medicine, seemingly, at all: Adidas shoes and Kentucky Fried Chicken—yet they led into a story about the importance of listening carefully to patients, for they will often tell you exactly what you need to know.

Von Hoff's story begins in 1995. A researcher, Gerald "Jerry" B. Grindey, who worked for Eli Lilly pharmaceutical company, told Von Hoff about a drug he had developed that seemed effective in shrinking tumors for lung and pancreatic cancers in animals. Grindey wanted to try the drug—called gemcitabine—in humans, and Von Hoff was able to get it approved for use in patients for a Phase I trial. This is very often exactly how the bench-to-bedside translation works. A researcher has a substance that shows interesting qualities and needs to find a patient sample to test it out; Von Hoff and TGen are frequent destinations for researchers. Based on the animal studies, Von Hoff established a dosage to try on a patient—I'll call him Jim—and, as is often the case, the drug caused harmful side effects, including what may have been a heart attack. After Jim recovered, Von Hoff reduced the dosage and tried gemcitabine on him again. Changing dosage of an experimental drug is common practice.

Jim was at the Veteran's Administration Hospital in San Antonio, where Von Hoff's laboratory was then located. Von Hoff remembered that he had been out of town for a while—colleagues had been following Jim on a daily basis—and that when he finally returned to see Jim, his wife complained. "You are late, Dr. Von Hoff. Twenty minutes!"

"I know," Von Hoff admitted. "I'm sorry."

"We are in a hurry today," the woman said. "Jim doesn't want to miss the Kentucky Fried Chicken. We like to be there when they open and get the first bucket that comes out of the fryer."

Ordinarily, said Von Hoff, he would have dismissed these comments as idle friendly chatter and moved directly into a physical examination, but this information struck him as odd. First of all, he pointeded out, a person with pancreatic cancer has serious fatty food intolerance: "They can't even drive by Kentucky Fried Chicken without getting sicker than they are, if that is even possible. And they lose weight—pounds melt away—because they can't eat anything." And yet, when Von Hoff glanced down at the patient's chart he was astounded to discover that Jim had gained seventeen pounds in two weeks.

"Jim," the wife told him, "eats a couple of buckets of chicken a day."

"Is that right?" Von Hoff said. He looked down at his patient's feet. "New shoes?" Von Hoff asked, motioning to the very white, unmarked Adidas track shoes.

"We actually walk to Kentucky Fried Chicken every day from the hospital. Jim's got energy like crazy."

Which is how Dr. Von Hoff first came to realize that gemcitabine was working in the first human patient in which it was ever tried. "We got a CT scan. Sure enough, his tumor was smaller."

So gemcitabine did work—or at the very least, it extended the lives of patients suffering from pancreatic cancer longer than any other drug. Not for all patients, Von Hoff went on to explain—and it was not the home-run cure that scientists hope for. But it was effective first-line therapeutic chemotherapy—the most helpful agent developed to that point to reduce the tumor's size and keep patients alive longer.

So how does this play out for patients? First of all, standard treatment for cancer usually means radiation or chemotherapy—toxic agents—like shotgun blasts or bombs that detonate on the tumor and everywhere else, more or less, in a patient's body. But drugs and protocols have been developed, or can be developed, that pinpoint a problem and work effectively on certain types of cancer—sometimes, Von Hoff added. He paused to shake his head and say the word again: *sometimes*.

Prediction is what doctors want to be able to do: to learn enough through research, into protein biomarkers, for example, to be able to tell patients the truth—and to give them hope, especially when the cancer is caught in time or when the patient and doctor are lucky enough to understand the tumor and to be able to make a medication match. Often, however, prediction is impossible. As I have pointed out before, and as Von Hoff has stressed, so much of what is accomplished in science is trial and error—and the emphasis, Von Hoff joked, may often be on error.

"So you take platinum, as an example." This story played out in a laboratory at Michigan State University, where scientists were attempting to increase the growth rate of bacteria using electricity. A young scientist working on the project came into the laboratory one morning and discovered that, contrary to expectation, the bacteria had stopped multiplying.

Annoyed, she blamed herself for turning off the electricity—a stupid oversight—but the lead investigator on the project, her supervisor, realized that something else had occurred. The electrodes creating the electrical field were connected, quite correctly, and turned on. It seemed, rather, that the bacteria had been poisoned by something emanating out of one of the electrodes. They realized that the electrode contained platinum, and ran tests to confirm that was the significant factor that had killed the bacteria. Then they started to think: if platinum killed bacteria, they asked themselves, what else might it kill? How about cancer cells?

"They tried out the drug cisplatin, which contained platinum," Von Hoff said, "and what do you think happened?"

At first, nothing happened; they tested the drug to no effect against a diversity of tumors—with the exception of a testicular cancer tumor, where it was quite effective. Not that it worked perfectly right from the start, but gradually an investigator in Indiana, Dr. Lawrence Einhorn, got it right by combining it with a couple of other drugs. Over the years the cisplatin-based drug combinations have been refined, just as Von Hoff had refined the dosage of gemcitabine for his KFC patient, and now yield remarkable results targeting the weakness in the specific tumor. The current cure rate for testicular cancer in all but the most advanced cases is in the neighborhood of 95%. Initially, the possibility of long-term survival for Lance Armstrong, perhaps the most famous cisplatin recipient, was estimated at no better than 50%. But platinum—cisplatin—led to seven first-place finishes in the Tour de France. Platinum targeted the context of vulnerability in one strain of testicular cancer.

Cisplatin, by the way, has another name, popular with nurses on oncology floors: "cisflatten." It turns out cisplatin, although therapeutic, causes overwhelming queasiness and nausea that literally knock patients, dry-heaving, to the ground, which is why the nurses call it "cisflatten"—it flattens their patients. The average cisplatin patient on a hospital ward will vomit a dozen times a day. They can be recognized anywhere in the hospital by the barf buckets they carry around wherever they wander—and pretty soon there's nothing left to vomit, except air, which doesn't stop the nausea for a minute. Thus, dry-heaving. For a while, cisplatin was thought to be a miracle cure-all cancer drug, and it was used for all sorts of tumors, so there were many "cisflatten" casualties in many different oncology wards.

Getting the drugs with the most potential to try on tumors is one challenge in the research process, but finding viable tumors is also a complicated process. Many laboratories like TGen have formed collaborations with physicians and surgeons at hospitals who collect and biopsy tumors from patients and then share the samples. The tumors are clinically annotated, which means that the patient's background, age, the rate of metastasis and other distinguishing points are noted. The researcher will want to determine how one tumor differs from another. The researcher will also attempt to isolate the biomarkers, if any, associated with the tumor. So the entire process leading from personalization to precision is tedious—there's no shortcut. Find a substance, find a tumor—and see how they dance with one another. This goes on day and night, haphazardly, as patients wait for miracles—or die without them.

Because he is dealing with patients at the ends of their lives, and with families at the ends of their ropes, Von Hoff works extra hard to tell stories and use examples so that his patients and their families can understand the complicated science he is attempting to develop. He also works hard to relax his patients and make them feel comfortable and supported—and he keeps them on their toes. This is part and parcel of personalized medicine. Part of the game when dealing with patients in trauma is understanding, and another equally important part is trust. Von Hoff works hard for his patients scientifically and spiritually, which is the way all doctors should operate.

Patients arriving at the clinic, for example—and some arrive unannounced—might assume that they've gotten off on the wrong floor, "either the pediatrics ward or the animal lab," Von Hoff joked, because a menagerie of animals awaits them as they step off the elevator. The animals are also part of personalizing personalized medicine.

"There is something magic about stuffed animals," said Von Hoff. "I've just always felt that there's some special comfort associated with them. I've had many patients give me stuffed animals—gigantic beasts—over the years as gifts, and the animals always made me smile. But they have really special meaning. You take my mother-in-law. She lived a good long life, but near the end she had dementia. The family had a collie way back when, named Lucky. Now this woman didn't know where she was at all—or who she was—or who I was. But one day I bought her a nice big collie—a really good-looking stuffed animal—and I walked in with that dog and she said right away, 'Lucky.' It was pretty remarkable. That's personalized medicine."

On a whim one day a few years ago, Von Hoff went into a local toy store and bought every large stuffed animal in the place. "Teddy bears," he said, "the Energizer Bunny—and golden retrievers. Anything and everything they had. I went to the clinic and gave them to a couple of patients, and it was amazing. They couldn't believe somebody gave them something so precious. The whole place changed.

"You put a dog in their midst, I mean a good-looking stuffed animal, and they immediately start talking about the fact that they had a dog some time in their past, and then lost the dog, the dog died, ran away—on and on—whatever. You connect. It is something else for patients to talk about rather than 'I got the bad cancer, it's eating my chest wall away, it stinks and I can't be near anybody.' Stuffed animals are nonjudgmental. They're sitting there watching the patients get an infusion, and you can see people look up and eyeball them and they just laugh. It really is disarming.

"So I just started getting more animals for our menagerie," said Von Hoff, launching into a chanting liturgy. "I got zebras, baby zebras and big zebras. I got baby giraffes and regular giraffes. I got Clydesdales. I got pandas. I got hedgehogs and an aardvark a guy brought from South Africa. I'd never seen a stuffed aardvark before. I got warthogs. It's a real zoo—very personalized because we got every animal known to mankind. I've got this chimp, beautiful chimp, and one of the nurses made a white coat for it, so when I come in to see a patient, I say 'I want to introduce you to my consultant here' and so it's amazing because people get off, and they break out laughing because they're scared. But my consultant takes the edge off for people—it helps them go forward."

So establishing the context of vulnerability and practicing personalized medicine is a three-stage affair, beginning with listening to and understanding the patient. And then there is identifying the genomic configuration in a patient's tumor that makes it weak or susceptible. And then, the crucial next step: what guns are available to capitalize on this susceptibility?

It would be terrific—but much too elementary—if this process described the route to killing cancer. Von Hoff uses a baseball metaphor to describe the dream: Check the DNA and then check the place of birth—that is first base. Next, examine the tumor for its Achilles heel—second base. Find an agent that will murder it—third base. And then go on and live a happy life—home run!

Alas, the game can't often be played that way. This has been the problem with genetics and personalized medicine from the very beginning—the idea that one disease can be traced to only one gene, which could then be taken out with one intervention. Unfortunately, the more scientists learn, the less this seems to be the case: there are perhaps twenty or thirty or more genes that connect with Alzheimer's, for example, and perhaps nearly as many for tumors.

For another thing, a tumor may have multiple weaknesses. Instead of one genetic link to cancer maybe there are a dozen. The best anyone can hope for is to find a corresponding compound for one of the contexts of vulnerability in the tumor. Then you can perhaps extend the patient's life until other agents are discovered and developed for other points of vulnerability in the tumor. And it may well happen that combinations or regimens of drugs—cocktails, so to speak, devised in the TGen laboratory—will be even more effective than the single agent being used, and perhaps cause fewer side effects over the years.

So, first you find the weakness in the tumor and then you find a drug that can affect the weakness. Like the sniper: take it out. This sounds simple, although it is not. Simple turns out to be convoluted and complex. A good example of how this works, sounding simple but turning complex, has to do with sheep. Not just any sheep—but cyclops sheep, sheep with only one eye.

CHAPTER 11:
THE HEDGEHOG

The story begins in the early 1950s in Idaho: Shepherds noticed that some of their sheep were giving birth to lambs with defects, underdeveloped brains and, most noticeably, only one eye in the middle of the forehead. The shepherds were concerned enough to reach out to the US Department of Agriculture to try to discover was happening. One scientist, Lynn James, was curious about what could be causing such weirdness, but was stumped. With a colleague, Richard Keeler, James studied the phenomenon for years without an answer, until he become so perplexed—and perhaps obsessed—that he summered with sheep in the mountains of Idaho for three consecutive years, to observe them, studying their feeding and grazing patterns. James eventually came up with the answer. He noticed that the sheep, while grazing, ingested large amounts of a large plant called corn lily, with green leaves and thick feathery flowers. So he and Keeler looked into the make-up of the corn lily and eventually determined that it contained a poisonous compound that blocks a chain of biochemical reactions important to embryonic development, disconnecting a pathway that sends signals to a sheep's embryos to develop two eyes rather than one. When James and Keeler (along with colleagues Wayne Bins and Lew Dell Balls) published their findings about this phenomenon in *Cancer Research* in 1968, they dubbed the compound "cyclopamine."

This discovery was interesting, but the researchers could never figure out exactly what was going on, and how cyclopamine caused sheep birth defects. Researcher Philip Beachy at Johns Hopkins University finally figured it out—twenty-five years later. Beachy also discovered that even people could be victims of such mutations.

There's a genetic pathway, called "the Sonic hedgehog" (named after Sega's elusive video game character), which, among other things, is a key component to embryonic development. Cyclopamine blocks the function of the Sonic hedgehog pathway. Subsequent researchers such as Jill Helms, who led a team at UC San Francisco and has since moved on to Stanford, discovered that babies with a faulty Sonic hedgehog pathway are born with holoprosencephaly, or HPE, a condition in which the child's brain fails to divide into two hemispheres in utero. These children have a wide range of disabilities, from severe mental retardation or an inability to speak to mild learning disorders. Facial defects can range from a cleft lip or a single front tooth to having just one eye in the center of the head. Other research demonstrated that abnormal activation in the Sonic hedgehog pathway could lead to cancers of the skin, prostate, lung and pancreas. Researchers working independently at Stanford and at the University of California, San Francisco, made separate but corresponding links, connecting basal skin cancer and a brain cancer called medulloblastoma, which usually afflicts children, to defects in the Sonic hedgehog pathway and related genes.

Beachy and his colleagues realized that cyclopamine could be used as kind of an off switch for abnormal activation in the Sonic hedgehog pathway. Also actively working in this area, Jingwu Xie, a scientist who is currently at the Herman B. Wells Center for Pediatric Research at Indiana University School of Medicine, conducted an experiment that marked the first successful drug treatment in animals of the most common cancer to afflict human beings—the skin cancer known as basal cell carcinoma (BCC). Xie spiked drinking water with cyclopamine and gave it to laboratory mice with BCC with dramatic results, demonstrating that the compound would significantly shrink existing tumors and prevent new tumors from developing.

Daniel Von Hoff was instrumental in taking this idea to the next step—Phase I trials, which are open to patients who have not responded to available standard therapies and have a life expectancy of no more than twelve weeks. Many patients, of course, live longer—or don't even survive the twelve-week estimate. Von Hoff learned that the pharmaceutical company Genentech had developed a cyclopamine-based drug, which it was calling GDC 0449, and he was able to get a supply. Here is another obstacle in personalized medicine that is not particularly well known or understood, and it concerns the changing role of the physician—or in this case the physician-scientist. Knowing what drugs are in development—and potentially available—is a full-time job. There are thousands of researchers in every corner of the world working in laboratories experimenting with new compounds—some of which have great promise.

Other than being an excellent clinician, Von Hoff is a notorious multitasker and a man constantly on the move. He stays on top of the literature, journal articles reporting on new developments, and simultaneously fosters good relationships with pharmaceutical companies. These days, scientists cozying up with big drug companies are often put under the microscope—the relationships can lead to conflicts of interest and suspicion because successful clinical trials can mean millions more in research money to the scientist and billions to the corporation. But this line of communication between the physician and the corporate laboratory is vital. And while the scientists need the drug to do their research and help their patients, the pharmaceutical companies need the clinician to move their product into human trials. This is where TGen and Von Hoff have an advantage.

Von Hoff can carefully select patients, matching drugs to particular tumors, as was case with the thirty-three patients he enrolled in the trial of GDC 0449. The first person to use 0449 had been in the TGen system, waiting for something to emerge that might help him. Jerry Coffman, a retired Phoenix city employee, had basal cell carcinoma that "had run amok," he said. Often caused by overexposure to the sun, basal cell skin cancers affect approximately a million Americans a year. Most are treated successfully with minor surgery, but in some patients, like Coffman, the cancer goes crazy. Coffman had been treated for basal cell carcinoma for seventeen years, undergoing lung surgery, three rounds of radiation and an unsuccessful experimental treatment. Von Hoff was on the case for Coffman, whom he told: "Hang on for six more months and I might be able to help you." Coffman knew he was dying, but he fought to stay alive for one more therapy. Every day, he said, he felt himself slipping, but you find hidden and unexpected resources when you have hope.

Meanwhile, around the same time Coffman was fighting to stay alive, Marie Petrini of Boulder, Colorado, had pretty much received her death sentence. In 1994, her ophthalmologist had noticed a small growth in her right eye. "I don't like the way that looks," he said. "We will have to keep watching it." Later the same year, she discovered that her eye contained a melanoma tumor, which was growing and spreading. The eye was removed and her doctor assured her that her worries were over—which they were, for thirteen years. But then an X-ray during a bout with pneumonia revealed a suspicious-looking lesion on a small lobe of her liver. A biopsy led to a diagnosis of melanoma, cancer that came from her eye. "A terrible shock," she said, "thirteen years later. No symptoms until then, suddenly everything bad happens. But that is how cancer goes." She went to the Mayo Clinic in Minnesota for help, and they put her in a clinical trial with a regimen of two medications, Abraxane and Carboplatin. It worked for nearly a year. "You know how chemo goes—severe hair loss, your whole body terribly abused." But she held on. And then, "I became allergic to Abraxane. Just like that. Nobody knew why."

As a last resort, surgeons opened her up, with hopes of excising the tumor, but the cancer was more or less everywhere. They closed her up, and she went home, ostensibly to die. But her husband telephoned TGen. Did they have anything that could help her? There are more than thirty experimental drugs in Phase I trials at TGen at any given time, and most of them don't have names. "I got a drug with a number," Petrini said. "E6201—whatever that is. But because of that number I have been alive a year longer than I ever imagined."

Coffman's life was eventually extended by the medication that blocked the hedgehog pathway, while Petrini's E6201 seemed to block what is called a "driver gene"—a mutation that seems prevalent in melanoma cancer. Half a dozen years ago, British scientists analyzing hundreds of tumor samples discovered that the same mutated gene, called *BRAF*, was present in more than half of the melanomas they studied. So if scientists could target and stop this driver gene, they might be able to stop melanoma. Lives could be saved; miracles could happen. E6201, it turned out, did exactly this—and it was effective for Marie Petrini's liver cancer. There are other *BRAF* inhibitors being developed by pharmaceutical companies and tested in medical centers in the United States and abroad. The idea of personalizing or "targeting" is catching on.

Interestingly, physicians conducting Phase I trials do not always target patients because of their type of cancer. The drugs like E6210 or 0449 are mysterious—sometimes magic bullets, but sometimes duds. While Phase I is ostensibly to test for toxicity, it is hard to predict what these drugs might do, how they will perform. E6201 helped Petrini with her liver cancer, though scientists at TGen had originally theorized that it would be most effective with leukemia patients.

Petrini remembered sitting in the waiting room in Scottsdale one day, waiting for her E6201 infusion. Her husband commented that a bunch of the nurses and doctors had congregated in an adjacent room. He was guessing that there was an important meeting going on there at the moment. "But then they all came out of the room and Dawn, the nurse who schedules appointments, was leading the way holding a cake with a candle on it and one year written on it—to me. I had lived on E6201 for one year. Happy anniversary."

While progress with E6201 and 0449 is miraculous, said Von Hoff, the bigger challenge, the most awesome part of working with sudden-death patients, is to keep patients alive long enough to help them. Basal cell, said Von Hoff, referring back to Coffman, can be "god-awful." It is usually removed surgically, but in the case of Coffman—the first patient to receive 0449—the cancer was eroding his face, and surgery was not possible. Immediately after he received the first dose of 0449, the tumors began to regress. "It was gone in four months!" Von Hoff exclaimed. Coffman's cancer had metastasized to his liver, bones and lung, but those tumors shrank dramatically, too. Coffman gained mobility—he had been nearly bedbound—and was working out in a local gym twice a week. He, too, might have purchased Adidas shoes.

The second patient to get 0449 had a horrendous pus-inducing scar on his ear that disappeared. The third patient to receive the drug was losing his ear; it was being eaten away by cancer, but it immediately began to regenerate. A fourth patient was losing his lungs—and they too regenerated. "It was a miracle," said Von Hoff. As often happens, as with Petrini, drugs targeted for one purpose are also discovered through trial and error to work on other tumors. Drug 0449 was also given to a twenty-six-year-old patient with brain cancer, who had a dramatic positive response. Although results are positive and hopeful, more testing and larger trials are required before 0449 can be commercialized.

In the meantime, Von Hoff continues to develop new treatment regimens, and enjoys occasional success stories, however fleeting some turn out to be.

Finding a cure is a process—slow and steady, one small success building on another. For example, Von Hoff has had a long and loving relationship with gemcitabine. Up until 2010, it had been the only drug that ever improved survival for patients with pancreatic cancer. "And it is a very gentle drug, as well. Most people can take the drug and keep on working." Recently, a group of French researchers have developed a four-drug chemotherapy regimen, Folfirinox, that has a better survival rate than gemcitabine alone. Von Hoff is now working on a regimen combining both drugs.

Gemcitabine is also now being combined with Abraxane—a combination that is extending life in many patients for six months to a year, and even longer. One patient Von Hoff recently treated, a seventy-nine-year-old man newly diagnosed with metastatic cancer of the pancreas, came to Scottsdale circling the drain, so to speak: "had a belly full of fluid, legs were swollen," and his prognosis was probably less than six months. But with this new regimen, he survived longer than he would have otherwise. He made it to his eightieth birthday, which was his goal: his last hurrah in life. His kids threw a big surprise party; he danced with his wife all night. He died not long after, but he had a good six months with real quality of life.

Some people may not think that this is such a good thing. The suffering, they would contend, may not be worth the final achievement, the brief extension of life. And then there's the expense of prolonging life. But there are those who cling to life—and who see some value in the contribution of those lives to science. Jim, the KFC patient, died within two years, but his contribution to science—the first patient to receive and respond positively to gemcitabine—was crucial. And while gemcitabine is clearly not the cure for pancreatic cancer that Von Hoff is seeking, it prolongs patients' lives with hopes that a cure or a better life-extending medication will be developed. Von Hoff urged Jerry Coffman to hang on and he would try to find something to keep his patient going—and he did, though Jerry also died within two years. One could say that this was a waste—that Jim and Jerry were destined to die, and that our scarce resources could have been redirected to a more positive or productive use—but who can make such judgments?

Patients at this stage of their cancer care, said Von Hoff, are very realistic. They've come to terms. "They know what I know—they are informed. And they are aware that we are living in a time when any of our new drugs could be the breakthrough in a certain disease and tumor type. We have seen this with the basal cell cancer, the hedgehog. We see this with the melanoma, and the good thing is we see this earlier and earlier. But it is all so complicated. The tasks are overwhelming—and the odds are always against us."

For example, it isn't that the combination of gemcitabine and Abraxane is more effective than gemcitabine alone in interfering with the growth of the tumor, says Von Hoff. The drug regimen actually serves different purposes—a complication that adds to the challenge of personalized medicine. Abraxane makes the gemcitabine work much better because it seems to cut through what is called the sTREM—anti-inflammatory tissue that blocks the cancer from receiving the chemotherapy—and allows the gemcitabine to attack the tumor directly.

"For instance, I had a CT scan a while ago, and the doctor said; 'Dan, what's that piece of wood doing in your elbow?' The memory came back to me. I was nine years old in Little League, but I was a terrible athlete. But once in a while if I kept swinging at the ball, I got a hit—I mean I hit the ball—and during one of those lucky moments, I was sliding into second base, and somehow I got a piece of wood in me—part of a broken bat, which at the time caused a staph infection." After a while, his immune system walled off the piece of wood, and it became part of who Von Hoff was. In the same way, the sTREM walls off the tumor and protects it, kind of like a watchdog—a guard dog protecting its master against foreign invaders.

Which brought Von Hoff back to his dual role of physician and scientist. Almost all of the patients who come to Scottsdale have already been treated with the tried-and-true traditional therapies—radiation, chemotherapy, whatever is available. They've often traveled far and wide, seeking help, unsuccessfully, and by the time they reach Von Hoff at Scottsdale, they are past the point of desperation in most cases and have begun to acclimate themselves to the idea that their time is short. But the possibility of making a contribution makes the journey more meaningful to the patient and, more importantly, to the friends and family surviving them.

CHAPTER 12:
FORGOTTEN CONSTITUENCY

At one point during his talk at the AAAS conference at the Arizona Biltmore, Leland Hartwell referred to the randomized clinical trial system for medical research, patient management and drug development. It is "a great approach," he allowed, but "insufficient for the problem," which, as he had previously outlined, challenged the government (the FDA), pharmaceutical companies and scientists to work together to develop and bring drugs to the marketplace more quickly. Hartwell made it clear that we have forgotten a valuable constituency in the bench-to-bedside process: patients.

"There is an increasingly important role for patients in this whole process . . . crucial," he emphasized, "to the future of medical science." As an example "of where we need to go," Hartwell referred to PatientsLikeMe, and its director of research and development, Paul Wicks, who happened to be in the audience that day. Although he was barely thirty years old at the time, Wicks had been involved as a researcher and patient advocate for more than one third of his short life—and unlike many advocates he was not, and had never been, a patient himself.

In 2002, as a twenty-two-year-old PhD student, Paul Wicks logged on to a message board for patients in the UK with amyotrophic lateral sclerosis—ALS, also known as Lou Gehrig's disease. Wicks's research focused on dementia in people with ALS, and the first thing he did upon logging on to the message board was to get in a fight. As it happened, the patients in the online forum were discussing the uselessness of Wicks's own research project.

But soon Wicks gained the trust of the ALS online community. The message board had begun as part of an innovative research project at King's College Hospital in London, where Wicks was studying. This was one of the first virtual support groups ever to be sponsored by a hospital. Eventually Wicks took responsibility for moderating the online discussion among patients. It was, he discovered, something like being made the vicar of a small village.

The online community, which was called Build UK, had been set up for people with muscular neuron disease and related syndromes; confined to wheelchairs, these patients could not attend support-group meetings at the hospital. But Wicks soon discovered that Build UK delivered far more than the usual support group held in a hospital basement. The online message board felt like a town, a place where people lived. The patients dropped into the website at all hours of the day and night; they considered each other close friends even though most of them had never met in person; and they came from all over the world to discuss their rare diseases.

Today, millions of people have flocked to virtual worlds where they can learn about their illnesses. According to a recent Pew Internet & American Life survey, 60% of Americans research their health problems online and use the Internet to check their symptoms; 7% of adults have gotten health information from social-networking sites.

Wicks, one of the first medical researchers to embrace social networks, believes that they will revolutionize medicine. As he sees it, the millions of patients who are gathering online can become a powerful engine for medical innovation; this is especially true when people are sorted carefully into groups that reflect their genetic mutations and disease subtypes. Wicks is a leading practitioner of research that is blazingly fast, cheap and nuanced. Already, his Internet-based investigations—data crunching, really—have led to new insights about rare syndromes. Questions that would have once taken a decade to answer can now take a matter of months.

For Wicks, unlike many scientists these days, new research methods grew out of a muddle of truck exhaust and road maps. In 2002 he started driving a lot, crisscrossing the roads of Britain to interview patients with ALS. The people he studied couldn't walk, and they were scattered all over the country. "You can't ask someone who's disabled, 'Would you mind popping down for six hours of neuropsychology tests in South London, please?'" Wicks explains. That's why he went to the patients' houses. Now that computers and the Internet are ubiquitous, especially in Western countries, Wicks's work would not be so travel intensive, but his crusade back then was necessary.

As he rang doorbells, sat in living rooms and drank lots of tea, he became an expert in all the ways that these patients were underserved by the British medical system. Some wheelchair-bound people lived in apartments three flights above the street; they had become prisoners in their own homes. Most shameful was the way patients had been diagnosed incorrectly or given very poor information. At that time, Wicks was a baby-faced graduate student and rabid science-fiction fan. He peppered his conversation with references to *Star Wars*, *The Matrix* and Harry Potter; he himself looked young enough to be enrolled at Hogwarts. But now he was spending hours in the homes of dying people, and he had to help them work through problems that were all too real. Wicks would show up to administer a cognitive test and, as he answered the patients' questions about the disease, would sometimes end up helping the patient prepare for the grim consequences of the illness.

He discovered several patients who thought they had ALS, when in fact they suffered from the rarer progressive muscular atrophy (PMA) subtype of the disease, which affects only the lower part of the body. (ALS affects the entire body.) One patient, for instance, wanted to know why he was still alive, five years after being told he should be dead. Wicks told him the details of this obscure diagnosis: the man actually had PMA and might live another decade. The patient had never heard of his own disease, and there were no pamphlets or online articles about the condition—until Wicks wrote one.

"I would invariably end up drawing the same diagram over and over. 'Here's your upper motion neurons.' 'Here's your lower motion neurons.' 'Here's what's affected.' People didn't know," Wicks says.

The consequences of misdiagnosis could be devastating. One lady, believing that she had only a year and a half to live, sold her house and took her family on a trip around the world. She went on to live another twenty-six years, with no savings and no house.

As Wicks spent more time with patients, he became interested in a question far outside his PhD research. He was shocked that patients had such weak ties to their hospitals. In certain obvious ways, this led to the neglect of those who were housebound. But Wicks also began to understand that the isolated patients experienced another kind of neglect; they were understudied. Researchers, for the most part, can only recruit subjects who can travel to a research center. They often study the most typical cases, rather than the outliers. This is one reason why Dr. Von Hoff opens the doors at TGen to all comers, to try to cast the widest possible net. But most people who are really sick and dying can't travel for treatment, even if the treatment itself is free. And so certain diseases remain mysterious, with no treatments or cures on the horizon.

Wicks wondered how the wheelchair-bound patients could be pulled into the loop. It didn't occur to him, at first, that the answer to many of these problems might be the Internet. But the solution presented itself when he took over Build UK.

The online community flourished, and Wicks became excited about the possibilities. A housebound California patient with one rare form of ALS could finally chat with his counterpart in Calcutta. And now Wicks could field questions from all of these people at once, running off to geneticists or gynecologists in the hospital when he himself did not have the answer. Instead of talking with one patient at a time, he could deliver information to an entire community.

Wicks suspected he'd just discovered one of the most important medical tools of the future. Even while he was educating patients, they were educating him. He lived among them, in their virtual town, like an ethnographer. He had become a citizen of their country.

But, of course, Internet communities come with their own set of problems. And the site that Wicks administered suffered from the kinds of rumors and flame wars typical of any online discussion board. What particularly bothered Wicks was the speed with which snake oil could spread through an online community of patients desperate for a treatment. When one patient discovered a "miracle cure"—from snake venom to wasp stings to stem cells—other people would pick up the idea and want to try it. Wicks warned members away from the most dangerous nostrums, but he was vastly outnumbered. And the patients invariably shouted him down. "I would say, 'I think that's not going to work.' And they would say, 'Oh, that's just because you're a mainstream scientist, you don't care about us,' or 'You're in the pocket of Big Pharma,'" he recalls.

At one point, a truly terrible idea took hold among the community members. This "cure" involved flying to China, paying as much as $20,000 and then submitting to an operation touted as a stem-cell transplant. A Chinese "doctor" would drill two holes in the patient's skull and then inject various substances in the brain and spinal cord. Afterward, the patient would be rehabilitated with traditional Chinese medicine, physiotherapy and cupping. Reports from the hospital suggested poor hygiene standards, a major concern for such vulnerable patients.

"I tried dozens of times to persuade people this was not going to work," Wicks recounts. It was infuriating that he, a medical professional, could not talk patients out of dangerous treatment. Eventually, one of the members of the online community actually flew to China and submitted himself to the hustlers. The unfortunate patient returned home with meningitis, diarrhea and a surgical instrument embedded in his neck. The sick man wrote up his gruesome story and posted it on the Web, warning others. That patient's story then became Wicks's strongest piece of counterevidence, and he urged ALS professionals to show it to any patients considering the trip to China. From that moment on, Wicks could immediately respond to any discussion of the "miracle cure" by reposting the horror story. Patients were immediately convinced by the message from a peer.

Wicks had learned a crucial lesson: though patients were often suspicious of the medical community, they trusted one another absolutely. The trick, then, would be to push patients themselves to become astute analyzers of data, so that they could amplify good information and dispel rumors. That is, Wicks began to see how he could organize the community so that it became smarter. With his love of imaginary worlds, he began to think of these online sites as cities that could be designed around the needs of the inhabitants.

He'd also begun to understand just how vulnerable these online worlds could be—particularly because the hospitals' administrators viewed them as a side project to be funded on the cheap. The Kings College website for ALS patients ran on a shoestring, and so did most of the other patient communities. One of the biggest of these online meeting places, called Brain Talk, catered to 50,000 people with neurological disorders and was, at its launch, associated with Massachusetts General Hospital and Harvard. One day in July 2006, a few years after the research funding had dried up, the unthinkable happened: the server crashed. The online community winked out of existence and disappeared for a month. Eventually, its domain name—braintalk.org—went on the auction block and was sold to the highest bidder.

When Brain Talk crashed, patients fled to Wicks's site. "I got a mass exodus of Americans," he remembers. The patients were desperate for a place to communicate. "This was before Facebook [was open to everyone]. There were no other networks," according to Wicks. "It was like when [the planet] Alderaan got destroyed in *Star Wars*. Suddenly 50,000 people have just disappeared off the Web." Wicks mourned Brain Talk, too. He'd helped manage conversations there; he'd been, in effect, one of the regents of that planet. And now all his work had vanished.

Wicks began exploring cyberspace, hoping to find a place where he—and patients—could settle in without fearing that all of their data would *poof* into nothingness. Beyond that, he envisioned an online community that was designed from the ground up in order to facilitate research. Patients would need to be funneled together into groups that would reveal something about their disease—for instance, they could be grouped together by their genetic mutations.

In 2006, Wicks discovered the brand-new PatientsLikeMe site. "I came to the website and it was like someone had taken my best dream and made it happen without me having to write a grant," he recalls. Soon, Wicks found himself with a full-time job at the company's headquarters in Cambridge, Massachusetts Now, finally, he had a chance to build the planet of his dreams.

CHAPTER 13:
PATIENTSLIKEME

PatientsLikeMe was the vision of a young man, Jamie Heywood, after his brother Stephen was diagnosed with ALS in 1998. As he talked about his brother's case with researchers, doctors and biotechnologists, Jamie began to understand how the medical world worked, and why it discriminates against people with certain diseases. Big Pharma tends to neglect rare illnesses because there is little profit in drugs tailored to a few thousand people.

At any point in drug trials, a pharmaceutical company financing research may decide that there is not a large enough population of potential patients—customers—to justify development of a particular drug, no matter how promising. To this point, drug companies have traditionally poured money into potential blockbuster drugs at the expense of the more targeted products with a smaller marketing-profit potential. The drug companies have been understandably resistant to changing this model. Why ruin a good thing? Blockbuster medications—one drug for many people—have been very profitable. Recently, driven by successful and profitable experiments such as with cisplatin, and by pressure from patients, physicians, scientists and the media, this blockbuster culture is slowly changing.

Still, some more rare illnesses receive far less attention. At the same time, the diseases are not entirely orphaned: academic researchers study rare syndromes, and university labs generate lots of ideas for the development of promising treatments. But that's where innovation often stops. There are few organizations that are willing to supply the funds to explore these ideas and to develop drugs. As Hartwell reminded the audience at the Biltmore, this has been an enduring problem in the medical world for decades. There has to be a way to speed up this process without sacrificing efficacy.

So Jamie Heywood and his family started up a foundation to do just that. The intention behind the ALS Therapy Development Institute (ALS TDI) was, in effect, to practice an extreme form of personalized medicine, since their goal was to save one man—and, of course, to benefit others along the way. A new drug can take a decade to develop, but the Heywoods' schedule—as well as the type of experts they hired and the research they sponsored—would be determined by the particulars of Stephen's disease.

It was an unusual way to pursue a cure, to say the least. Jamie liked to call it "guerilla science" because scientists would be forced to investigate familiar questions from new angles. The researchers had no choice but to innovate. And the foundation—run by a well-heeled family steeped in engineering—would operate in the nimble, highly caffeinated manner of a dot-com startup. With the help of Dr. Steve Gullans from the Harvard Medical School, the family developed a plan to test many of the drugs approved by the US Food and Drug Administration to see if any of them held promise for ALS. The experimental compounds would be given to lab mice that had been engineered to die of ALS within several months. Between 2001 and 2006, according to ALS TDI, the foundation "screened more potential therapeutics for ALS than all other research labs in the world combined."

But a cure, if it were to come, would not arrive soon enough for Stephen. Confined to a wheelchair, he scooted about his house, taking in nutrition through a feeding tube. His speech became so hard to understand that he switched to talking through a computer. He typed by shrugging his head to one side; the computer spoke for him in its robot voice. Stephen regarded his own life as a matter of engineering: to stay alive, and to continue communicating and moving, he would need the best machines available. Jamie Heywood, too, recognized just how grim the situation had become. "What if what we're doing here is impossible?" he asked.

So it was that Jamie Heywood threw himself into creating a brand new tool that patients could use to pool their knowledge about their diseases—not only about treatments and testing, but also about equipment and products. PatientsLikeMe—a social-networking website—launched in 2006. Stephen Heywood was its first member. But he did not have a chance to see the site grow. In November of 2006, Jamie posted an open letter to friends and family, letting everyone know that his brother had died.

Jamie did not allow his brother's passing to slow down his efforts; to the contrary, he was inspired by it and was now on a mission to save—or at least, improve—the lives of as many people as possible with data. His point was that data is as much a part of the effort to save lives as are our genes—a factor that many personalized-medicine advocates would not debate. Jamie had created what he calls the perfect tool for personalized medicine: a social-networking community that would give patients a way to see the fine grain of their disease, and thereby pursue a tailor-made treatment. A year after the site launched, CNN Money named PatientsLikeMe one of the fifteen companies that will change the world.

But how does one build a community that is designed to support patients and researchers alike? Wicks and his confreres at PatientsLikeMe had to figure out ever-finer ways to divide up illnesses. What we call multiple sclerosis, for instance, seems to be a collection of related illnesses with different origins and rates of progression. Some patients attribute their disease to certain environmental factors or infections. Other patients can't find an environmental trigger but have a family history of the illness. And the symptoms of MS vary wildly from person to person; neurologists say, "If you've seen one case of MS, you've seen one case of MS."

As a consultant to PatientsLikeMe, Wicks worked on designing the MS and Parkinson's disease communities, which meant encouraging members who joined the site to share useful information about their disease. "You would think that if you're talking with any patient with some disability then you could just ask, 'Are you currently using a wheelchair?' 'How far can you walk at the moment?' 'Can you bathe yourself?' That stuff is straightforward. But how frequently do you ask that question? What words do you use? Do you phrase it positively? Do you mean 'sometimes' or 'always' use a wheelchair? It's very complicated. So I would never advocate for saying users themselves can pull together a set of questions and it could be meaningful," Wicks said. The site itself would have to lead members through an analysis of their own illness, prompting them to think about questions that probably would not occur to them otherwise.

Now, Wicks needed a way to guide MS patients to divide themselves into groups—but what kind of groups? Because he'd been trained in a university system, Wicks said, he had assumed it would take several years and a small fortune for PatientsLikeMe to come up with a way to sort the MS patients into meaningful groups. The way these things are usually decided in academia is to fly a dozen experts to a hotel, form subcommittees and make plans for further discussion in a year's time. But Jamie Heywood pushed for the team to make sense of MS from a new perspective. They felt that the old way of doing things was as much about academic ritual as real work; they thought that with the right team, the important questions could be solved in a few hours.

At first, Wicks resisted this process. "At the time I said, 'No, absolutely not. We haven't been published. It's not rigorous enough.'" But in the end, that's how PatientsLikeMe designed its disease communities: by vigorous debate between smart people, fueled by a lot of caffeinated beverages. After a couple of new communities had been developed in this way, Wicks developed a process called DRIVE that guides researchers to "Define, Research, Innovate, Visualize and Execute" community designs.

The PatientsLikeMe site relies entirely on data collected by patients themselves. And that's one of its weaknesses, because people can be horribly unreliable when it comes to reporting on their own bodies. I discovered this firsthand when I set up my own Google Health record. When Google Health asked me to supply my weight, I lied, shaving off a few pounds. In fact, I didn't even realize that I was lying; at the time, I owned a broken scale that always gave me a weight that I liked. It was only later, when I stepped onto a scale at the gym, that I realized I'd reported my "fantasy weight" to Google Health. When it comes to our bodies, sometimes we see what we want.

On PatientsLikeMe, the members are guided every step of the way as they enter information, to make their self-reports as accurate as possible. They are encouraged to catalogue their symptoms, which are represented in medical language, on a stick-figure graphic of their body, and on a charted timeline. For instance, a patient who specifies that he has the progressive-relapsing form of MS might answer questions about possible problems with walking; his own body would then be represented by a red-legged stick figure, so that other patients can see his problems at a glance.

As part of their profiles on PatientsLikeMe, patients are also asked to enter information about the genes they carry. It's this genetic data that may offer the greatest insights for researchers. For instance, dozens of patients with ALS are getting tested for several specific mutations and are including some of that genetic data in their profiles. Chillingly, the research team at PatientsLikeMe can watch how the different mutations affect patients by monitoring their behavior on the site. Those who carry a mutation associated with rapid death from ALS tend to sign up, enter a lot of information and then stop logging in after a few months. Those with a far less deadly mutation, on the other hand, join the site and stick around for many years.

For years now, Wicks has listened in on these patients as they discuss the medical system that seems to hold them hostage. He's befriended many patients who are furious that clinical studies seem to be set up to advance the careers of academics rather than to benefit the sick. It is heart wrenching for a patient to enroll in a study and place his faith in an experimental drug, for example, only to learn that he'd been given a placebo. For someone with six months to live, that is cruel indeed.

It is not just the members of PatientsLikeMe who feel this way. *The Oncologist* reported in 2008 on a crisis in research: about half of all cancer studies fail to recruit enough patients to go forward. Quite simply, many sick people are defecting from academic research. Patients read the medical journals; they can sniff out the pointless studies. "They ask, 'Why is this drug being studied? We know from the mice it didn't work,'" Wicks said. "They don't really feel engaged in that dialogue, and that's dangerous for clinical trial recruitment." Lee Hartwell has observed that scientists are also prevented from acquiring valuable research information due to censoring. Scientific journals will inevitably publish only papers reporting successful studies. But Hartwell points out that there is much to be learned from studies that fail, "and we never hear about them."

Even as patients defect from traditional research, however, they are flocking online. Sites such as PatientsLikeMe, CureTogether and ACOR (an online cancer community) have no trouble attracting people who want to participate in trials. This allows for an entirely new form of medical research powered by a Wikipedia-like army of volunteers.

For instance, a few years ago, an Italian medical study published in the prestigious *Proceedings of the National Academy of Science* (PNAS) suggested that the drug lithium might slow the progression of ALS. The study was inconclusive, however, and it left patients in a quandary: Should they take lithium and risk suffering from side effects? Or should they skip the drug and lose out on its potential benefits? The designers of PatientsLikeMe decided to answer the question themselves. Their method of research would be cheap indeed. The site simply asked the patients who were taking lithium to report their dosages, blood-level readings and symptoms. More than 200 patients on lithium participated, and hundreds more who were not taking lithium formed a control group. Within just a few months, the patients had found their answer: lithium did not slow the progression of the disease in the PatientsLikeMe population.

Of course, this is not the kind of research that one normally sees in *The New England Journal of Medicine*. For one thing, the patients collected and reported their own data—a seat-of-the-pants method that is considered by some to be highly unreliable. Still, if the patients had taken part in a comparable academic study, they might have had to wait five or more years for the results to be published. Wicks has begun to view Internet-based studies like this as a challenge to the academic system. Why should funders back research that takes ten years to answer a question? Now, said Wicks, "You can answer that same question in an afternoon."

CHAPTER 14:
PATIENT WITH AN E

Of course, PatientsLikeMe is far from the only social networking site to bring patients together, and Jamie Heywood and Paul Wicks—as dedicated and passionate as they are—are not victims of disease. The patient experience is obviously different from the advocate's; it is more desperate, more crucial and pressing. More "real," as Dave deBronkart will tell you. In January 2007, deBronkart lay on an examining table as a technician rubbed a probe up and down his torso. On the monitor beside him, a black-and-white topography of deBronkart's insides rolled across the screen.

Only two weeks earlier, deBronkart had thought of himself as a healthy middle-aged guy with nothing to complain about but a tweaked shoulder. Then an X-ray on his bum shoulder revealed a mysterious shadow on his lung. After further testing, his doctors delivered the terrible news: deBronkart's lungs appeared to be dotted with metastatic cancer. It was likely that the disease had not started there. The original tumor could be hiding anywhere in deBronkart's body; his doctors would have to find it.

Now, in the ultrasound room, his wife leaned over to stare at the monitor. She'd been trained as a veterinarian, and had examined plenty of ultrasounds in her practice. In the black-and-white storm on the screen, she saw trouble. She told deBronkart she'd spotted a tumor in one of his kidneys. A few minutes later, deBronkart stood outside the ultrasound room and called his primary care physician, Dr. Danny Sands, who happened to be in California at the time. Sands is a part-time primary care physician and an expert in information technology. He immediately picked up. As soon as he heard Dave's voice, he knew the prognosis must be shockingly bad. Dave was sobbing. The two men had forged a friendship; now, Sands was devastated to learn that deBronkart might have one of the deadliest forms of cancer.

Days later, a biopsy confirmed the terrible diagnosis. When deBronkart learned the results, he sank into a chair, stared into the screen of his laptop and typed "kidney cancer" into Google. Clicking his way through page after page, he tried to find the shape of his new future. The medical sites all seemed to give the same verdict: "Outlook is bleak." "Prognosis is grim." But it was almost impossible to find the answer to the question burning in his mind: "What are my odds?" Finally he found a site that let him "score" his disease. He typed in all the particulars of his case. Out popped an answer: a median survival time of twenty-four weeks.

"That night was hell," deBronkart wrote later in his journal. "Never see another Christmas? Maybe not even see summer?" He was then a fifty-seven-year-old-high-tech marketer with a mellow voice and a whorl of salt-and-pepper hair. He marketed software for customers on the Internet, a job he loved. As an evening hobby, he sang baritone with a barbershop chorus and had recently started his own quartet. But now this happy existence seemed to have been yanked away by a clump of killer cells in his kidney.

A few days later, deBronkart sat in a consulting room with Danny Sands. The two men were kindred spirits, both of them fascinated with extending the reach of the Internet. Sands had coauthored the first published guidelines for the use of doctor-patient e-mail. At Beth Israel Deaconess in Boston, the doctor was part of a team that had pushed for computers in every medical examination—and pioneered the simple but unusual practice of turning the monitor toward the patient. Now Sands divided his time between seeing patients and working for Cisco Systems Internet Business Solutions Group.

That day, Sands scrawled out an unusual prescription on his pad: "acor.org." The Association of Cancer Online Resources happened to offer a particularly vibrant community of kidney cancer patients. That night, deBronkart joined the ACOR mailing list and began "lurking"—observing—for a couple of days, to see how an online community conducted itself. The www.acor.org website, according to deBrokart, is not pretty; it has no fancy graphics. What makes it special are the highly informed and generous people who gather there. "It ain't the platform; it's the people," he says, that makes an online community valuable. Finally, he worked up the courage to introduce himself. Within fifteen minutes, one of the members sent the name of the top kidney specialist in the country. Later, someone else on the list recommended that deBronkart try a treatment called high-dosage interleukin-2.

As it turned out, deBronkart's specialists agreed with the recommendation he'd received online; they, too, believed that interleukin-2, an immune-system booster, was his best hope. DeBronkart had to pass several hurdles to make his way into the clinical trial of the drug. Studies he found online showed that the drug worked its miracles for only 7–13% of kidney cancer patients; the rest of the patients were not helped. These terrible statistics loomed over the early days of his illness.

Still, he threw himself into pursuing the drug treatment, and into the role of managing his own career as a patient. For deBronkart, that meant employing his considerable skills as a geek. In his life before cancer, he'd been working at a company that made software for scheduling appointments on the Internet, and deBronkart had helped design (among other things) an online calendar that let dog owners set up grooming sessions at a Petco store.

DeBronkart had long recognized that doctors and hospitals lagged far behind other industries in their use of the Internet. Some medical offices had no website. The only way to reach them was to phone in and wait on hold. Often, he would then be told to call another office, and another. Booking one appointment could take an hour. The pure wastefulness of this system was appalling.

Luckily, though, deBronkart did not have to experience any of this hassle at his home hospital. Years earlier, he had chosen Beth Israel, partly because it was one of the first medical institutions to embrace the Web. Its online site, called PatientSite, lets patients make appointments and view some parts of their medical records. Created in 1999, the system had originally been, in part, the brainchild of Danny Sands. And now, Sands spearheads a movement that might potentially make the Internet the crown jewel of every medical practice, a tool that brings patients and doctors together as they collaborate to make sense of symptoms.

Sands spends a lot of time practicing medicine in the Internet cloud. Because he's also an IT expert, he practices as a doctor only part-time, seeing patients in his office on Fridays—and any time online. He works with patients as if they're colleagues—shooting them e-mails, responding to their questions, sending them links to medical studies or reading through the research they've sent to him.

"I want patients to be educated," he says. "I want them to be looking for information, even if they see it before I do. I encourage my patients to do that. I say, 'Here are some websites to check out.' We're working together to help the patient to get and stay healthy, rather than my trying to somehow foist health upon the patient. Furthermore, I don't believe that I'm the only person who knows things; the patient brings expertise to the table as well."

Sands points out that a new class of medical software is transforming the way doctors diagnose and prescribe. For those (like Sands) who use one, an electronic medical record can do far more than just store information. It can also catch errors, make suggestions about medications, point to relevant studies and crunch numbers.

Thus, physicians could truly become somewhat like airplane pilots, making decisions with the aid of specialized software that calculates the best path forward or alerts them to safety breaches. This kind of tool could revolutionize drug treatments. Every year, according to the US Department of Health and Human Services, prescription drugs cause more than 770,000 injuries and deaths in America. In many cases, the physician has done everything by the book, and the patient has responded badly to the standard dose of a one-size-fits-all medication. Many of our reactions to drugs—good, bad and deadly—can be traced to genetics. For example, in the case of warfarin, the blood-thinner, the ideal dose can vary by a factor of ten, depending on a patient's genetic make-up. Though a test for the "warfarin genes" is available right now, researchers are still figuring out how to use the results to fine-tune dosages. But within a year or two, this gene-based method of prescribing warfarin may become routine. Data will be the key to saving lives. Electronic medical records could contain an enormous amount of information about the patient's body, including the genes that determine the way the patient will metabolize common pills. Prescribing drugs could soon become a feat as complicated, and computerized, as landing a jet at JFK.

With Sands's encouragement, deBronkart had become an early adopter of the Beth Israel PatientSite in 2003. Following his cancer diagnosis in 2007, the Beth Israel website became his lifeline. He could write to Sands every day through a privacy-protected e-mail system; he could see his lab tests and access his radiology reports for CAT scans and X-rays. When he requested a medication from a doctor, it would be ready at his local pharmacy without a trip downtown to pick up the script. This convenience made all the difference to deBronkart as the winter deepened.

In February, a tumor developing in his femur had made it difficult to walk. He had to hobble around on a cane; eventually, he'd rely on a scooter. With characteristic élan, deBronkart delighted in zipping around on the machine and he even rehearsed with his barbershop chorus from its seat. Still, he had days when he struggled to get out of bed. It became all the more important to manage his care from his laptop.

Then, on June 18, 2007, deBronkart had good news. "It's official: I am an Interleukin Responder!" he typed into his journal, which was later published as a book. He'd endured several harrowing treatments with the drug, and now tests had showed that his hardships had paid off in a spectacular fashion. His cancer was vanishing. "The doctors' report today, evaluating last week's CAT scan, couldn't have been much better: the target lesions are 'dramatically smaller.' They're less than half their previous size," he reported.

Even as he celebrated his recovery, deBronkart wondered why he'd found such discouraging statistics during the early days of his treatment. And why did medical journals so often cite statistics based on old treatments, some of which weren't even used anymore? Why was it so hard to find information that reflected the latest research? If only he'd had that early on, he might have been spared the heartache of planning for his own death.

In his journal (which he originally posted online), he exhorted other patients to be suspicious of death sentences, especially since statistics tend to be hopelessly out of date by the time they're published in medical journals: "I'll never forget what it felt like to read . . . 'The outlook is grim.'" Patients, he railed, are often given incorrect information about their chances of survival. "Those stats just don't apply anymore. Ignore them," he urged.

In November 2007, only months after his recovery, deBronkart made this point to researchers when he attended a Kidney Cancer Patient Day in Boston. He filed into a meeting room at the Hyatt Regency, hobbling through a crowd of patients, clinicians and social workers. He used a metal cane now.

The first speaker, one of the world's top researchers of kidney cancer, showed a chart with the same statistics that appeared in every medical description of the illness. Those numbers made kidney cancer look like a death sentence. And yet, deBrokart was here, living proof of a different set of statistics.

When question time came, deBronkart found that the microphone had conveniently been placed right next to him, and he was the first to stand up, cane in hand. He started by thanking the doctor's team for saving him; "My tumors are reduced 80% from their original size." The room erupted into applause.

But then, deBronkart changed his tone. "The table you showed of median survival times—that's from the Kansas City Kidney Cancer database of cases collected through 1995, right? And none of today's treatments existed then, right?"

The doctor agreed.

"So," deBronkart said, "those figures have nothing to do with outcomes for someone who's diagnosed today, right?"

The expert said yes, this was true.

Then deBronkart burst out, "Well, I wish you guys would tell people that! These numbers scare people to death, and they're not current!"

Of course, deBronkart did understand why medical researchers used their dusty statistics; these numbers had been vetted, peer-reviewed and double-checked. Meanwhile, most brand-new studies have not been subjected to scrutiny. Still, in certain fields of medicine, the newer information is often much more valuable than the old—particularly to patients. When he leapt up to speak that day in Boston, deBronkart wanted desperately for the doctors and researchers to understand what numbers in medical journals mean to patients, and that these statistics haunt the prayers and the midnight terrors of real people.

After all, deBronkart himself had spent months on the brink of death; he'd been educated about the bad odds, but not about the scientific shortcomings of those same statistics. This brush with mortality had transformed him. He was brimming with a new passion to improve the healthcare system. And as a data guy, he could see so many ways to fix problems.

As a software jockey, deBronkart had a unique window on the many profound failures of the medical system. "If you went to check in online for a flight, and you got someone else's boarding pass, you would think this was ridiculous," he pointed out. "Modern data systems are reliable." And if a mistake does happen, you can easily fix it.

Not so in a hospital. In 2008, deBronkart learned this from firsthand experience. One day, as he was studying his electronic medical record on the Beth Israel system, he found a troubling error: an X-ray report from 2003 identified him as a female patient. Had a woman's X-ray been put into his file? And if so, how could he alert the unfortunate woman that he had her results? He called Beth Israel and tried to report the error. That's when he discovered that even his high-tech hospital had no mechanism for correcting scrambled medical files. Eventually, after months of back and forth, deBronkart determined that the X-ray had been his all along; it had simply been mislabeled. Still, he says, the hospital "had no process at all for dealing with a reported error. In fact the general consensus was, 'Why are you complaining at all?'"

Of course, most of us still can't catch these kinds of errors because we can't download our X-ray report or directly access much of our own medical data. Ideally, we would all be able to click into our hospital files as easily as we access our bank records. Additionally, most everyone agrees that the system should be standardized, so that the electronic file that works in a hospital in Boston can also be read by a doctor's office in Boise. But we're a long way from that ideal system. Most hospitals still use only paper files. Meanwhile, those hospitals and clinics that do offer cutting-edge digital systems exist in their own locked-in silos; files cannot be exchanged between hospitals in different parts of the country. That means that America's medical record keeping is hopelessly balkanized, a patchwork of incompatible programs.

Still, other countries are proving that universal systems can exist. In Denmark, almost every doctor, hospital and pharmacist participates in a national electronic system. Health professionals track patients from the examining table to the lab test to the drugstore. Nearly 100% of doctor visits since the year 2000 can be accessed on a computer—and, of course, patients control who can see their private data.

The bad news is this: it took a decade for the Danes to build their model system. It might take us just as long to build ours.

In the meantime, both deBronkart and Danny Sands recommend that all of us create and store our own electronic records; that way, at least we'll be able to keep our own information safe, even if we change hospitals. To create your own record, you need to use software designed for personal use rather than for hospitals. Currently, Google Health and Microsoft HealthVault are some of the best-known products in the still-obscure field of personally controlled health records.

It was soon after the Boston conference that deBronkart decided to become an evangelist for a wired healthcare system. Early in 2008, deBronkart discovered the term "e-patient." As soon as he heard the word, he knew he was one. Online, he adopted the handle E-Patient Dave. "My head blew apart," deBronkart said later, about the moment when he found his new name.

By 2009, he had become the most famous e-patient in the world. His is not exactly Britney Spears fame, but in the demimonde of healthcare IT, deBronkart has gathered his own fan base. He's now a frequent speaker at medical conferences and a witness at government and nonprofit policy meetings in Washington. He and Danny Sands appeared on a 2009 list of twenty top innovators in healthcare. Sands jokes that Dave deBronkart's transformation into E-Patient Dave had biblical overtones, and compares it to the moment in the Old Testament when Abram becomes Abraham. The extra "ah" in Abraham's name symbolizes a new relationship to God and community. E-Patient Dave, likewise, feels reborn into a new identity and into a new crusade. You can learn about his new life by reading his blog at www.epatientdave.com.

CHAPTER 15:
THE 7Q11.23 DUP GROUP

Geneticist Dr. Jonathan Berg first examined three-year-old Chloe Ruffino at Baylor University, where he was doing his residency. Before meeting Berg, Chloe's parents, Cherie and Louie, had consulted a number of pediatricians, both in private practice and at the Children's Hospital of Texas medical center, about their child's inability to speak. While some children take longer than others to begin to talk, the Ruffinos were certain that Chloe was far behind other children her age. Berg agreed and sent a DNA sample to the diagnostic lab at Baylor for a series of microarray tests. Microarray technology basically tests sample cells to find out what genes in each cell are expressed. In other words, it profiles the cells and the genes. Microarray also allows a researcher to compare healthy cells with diseased cells to see how they differ microscopically; for this reason, it is often used in cancer research.

Normally, people have two copies of most genes—one inherited from each parent. But sometimes a person can be born with fewer (one or none) or, in contrast, many more copies of a particular gene. Initially scientists believed that such "copy number variations" were thought to be very rare, but the more scientists learn the more surprised they are about how much of what they assumed was true is wrong. Today, scientists believe that at least 10% of human DNA may contain differences in copy number, which will sometimes (but not always) affect development and health. Berg told me that what happens because of the copy variations basically depends on which genes are involved and why they are important. We still have very little information about what the majority of genes do in our cells, he says. Some genes are very important for brain development and function; others are not.

In Chloe's case, Berg and his colleagues found that a region of the genome designated as 7q11.23, containing about twenty-five to thirty genes, had been duplicated. "When I first saw the patient, this same duplication had been reported only once in the medical literature, so we really had very little information for the family," Berg says. That initial report had actually made it into the *New England Journal of Medicine* because the duplication was the exact opposite of a deletion that causes a famous (at least by genetic syndrome standards) syndrome called Williams-Beuren syndrome (WBS), which may affect heath and development more severely than the 7q11.23 duplication.

It wasn't a surprise to Cherie and Louie Ruffino that Chloe had a legitimate problem with language development; they were well aware of that already, which was why they were working so hard to find help. But to receive a diagnosis of a disease with no name—no history, no research—and to consult with doctors who had absolutely no clue about what to do was startling and difficult to process. "I went home after learning about 7q11.23 duplication from Dr. Berg and cried," Cherie remembers. "How could it have happened?" That was the first question after the tears. "What did we do—or what did we have in our DNA or lack that caused such havoc? The best Dr. Berg could say was that at the time of conception the gene thought it wasn't there—it didn't read and comprehend that it was there, and so it actually recreated itself again, duplicated."

DNA, which is put together in long chains of amino particles, is often twisted and contorted inside a cell, so even though from a linear perspective the strands of DNA could stretch in a straight line, the bits of gene in a strand can and sometimes do connect to or feed off one another. This can lead to duplication or deletion in genes. Other inexplicable eccentricities of DNA are its tendencies to delete itself or, conversely, duplicate—spontaneously. You can't count on it to stay where it is—or how it is.

Francis Collins has another answer that he gives quite frequently: "The first law of the genome is that anything that can go wrong, will."

"Going wrong" may be applicable to what happened with the Ruffino family, though that might not be the best way to put it, scientifically. From the researcher's point of view, scientists were learning more and more every day—gathering information that can be confusing, on the one hand, but can also help us understand more about what makes us who we are.

Scientists have discovered, for example, that RNA, instead of merely aiding DNA with the synthesis of protein, may actually perform some functions once thought to be in the province of DNA only, and that "noncoding" (or "junk") DNA actually performs some crucial tasks, like protecting cells from viral attack. Particularly confounding is the fact that genes can be turned on and off, although we cannot predict when they are activated and deactivated and we do not know why this occurs. This on-off function, controlled by transcription factors, is often but not always inherited. Scientists have no clue why.

Why? How? These are the questions many parents are obsessed with—particularly when their children do not survive. They need closure, says Dr. Lane Rutledge, a pioneer in the field of genetics and pediatrics, who is now medical director of the Biochemical Genetics Laboratory, and director of clinical services, for the genetics department at the University of Alabama in Birmingham.

Rutledge, who began her medical career in pediatrics and child neurology, had, early on, a couple of patients who had "weird things happen to them, diseases that no one knew anything about. So I was told to admit these patients, treat them, go out and learn about them." She took a genetics fellowship and soon thereafter began practicing biochemical genetics and neurology, a path she has been following for twenty years now. Her patient population—the patients she follows—may be nearing 300, although some of the patients to whom she is the most committed are, as she puts it, "no longer with us. Meaning that they are dead."

A single mother with curly, flowing, gray hair and a raspy, crackling voice, Rutledge considers herself a physician and an investigator—a medical detective in the truest sense of the word. She picks up a pile of file folders at her desk and waves them in the air. "All of these patients," she says, "have something, some defect, some disease, some anomaly—something—I am trying to figure out." The patients carefully described and chronicled in these files can be divided into two groups: "Half of them are alive and the other half are dead." But dead or alive, Rutledge says, "I never give up finding out what happened to them."

She receives results from all of the newborn screenings in the hospital to compare with tissue or skin samples she has preserved from the patients she lost over the past twenty years. She uses hospital or donated money she begs or borrows for comparative testing. "Once the child is dead no one is going to pay for testing—even though the information I receive might save children in the future," she explains. Insurance companies, she says, are not helpful.

But Rutledge is relentless in her quest to understand what happened to her patients—and why. Once, a child came to the hospital all the way from Mississippi at four days old—"was sick as stink, acidotic as all get-out," she says in her gruff, southern, down-and-dirty twang. The child died within an hour of being admitted. Over the next year, she shipped his liver from lab to lab, from Ohio to Texas, for tests, until she discovered the cause of his death.

"What's the point in doing this?" she asks, rhetorically. "The child's life has been lost, I know. But now I have the information ready for the next patient with the same or similar symptoms. Or those patients may have siblings that may have anywhere from 25–50% chance of having the same thing."

To illustrate how such information gathered after the fact can be lifesaving, she discusses a recent case that involved one family. A child a few years old died from a genetic defect. Rutledge learned everything she could about what happened to the child and carefully considered what actions she might have taken had she known about the defect in advance. She was preparing herself to be ready to treat other children from this family more appropriately at birth—and beyond.

The mom got pregnant again, Rutledge explains. As soon as that baby was born "we put that baby on IV fluids—glucose." But that baby was not afflicted with the gene so the IV was removed. The same procedure was followed when the next baby from this same family was born. That baby did have the defect—and "because we treated that third child from the beginning, she never got as sick as her brother who died." The baby lived, in other words, despite the genetic defect because the medical team had been informed and prepared.

And of the mother with the child who died at four days, Rutledge explains: "She needed to know why her baby died—even if it was a year or even a decade later. Some people say, 'Why do you go and do this—searching for reasons when the patient is dying or dead? It is hopeless.' My response is, number one, it stops the search. Every parent with a child with a problem is obsessed with trying to figure out what it is, what happened to their baby. And sometimes there is a lot of guilt that maybe shouldn't be there. So you can tell them, 'Look, I have found a genetic cause for what happened. Nothing you did caused this.' And the second thing is, sometimes you can predict or at least tell people what they might expect in the future if they choose to have another child. People come in with many notions about why something has happened—from blaming themselves for what they did when pregnant, whatever you can imagine, to the phase of the moon, so parents need an answer, desire a sense of closure."

But where to go and what to do when the doctors say your child's disease is so new and mysterious that it has a weird code for a name, and they haven't the slightest idea what to do about it except to watch, wait and wonder?

As the Ruffinos were quickly discovering through Dr. Berg, the potential complications of genetic mutations are uncountable and perhaps unfathomable. The challenge for the Ruffinos was adjusting to the world that 7q11.23 duplication was presenting them.

Cherie and Louie, proactive people, started out by trying to gather information about 7q11.23 duplication. But there was nothing on the Internet; information didn't exist. They e-mailed Berg repeatedly because they knew that he was pursuing his research, and eventually gathered together several other cases of the same duplication. "We were able to draw some conclusions about the spectrum of phenotypes seen in patients with the 7q11.23 duplication," Berg says. "Interestingly, patients with the deletion"—Williams-Beuren syndrome— "and duplication seem to have some contrasting characteristics: relative strength of language in the deletion patients and severe language impairment in the duplication patients; outgoing personality in the deletion patients and autistic behaviors in some duplication patients. It isn't an exact inverse phenotype, but scientists who are really interested in language development and human behavior have found this pair of syndromes quite interesting."

The genetic causal chain is difficult to decipher. "We have a younger daughter, and she came out of the womb talking," says Cherie. The Ruffinos have been tested for 7q11.23 duplication, and neither is a carrier. Chloe is the first affected person in the family. Cherie speculates that Chloe will be able to pass the duplication on, so, she says, "When she gets to a time later in life, if she should be of an independent status and elects to start a family, that is going to be a conversation we are going to have to have with her, that this is what Mom and Dad went through and we will help you get through it, but I just want you to know what the future may bring. Having a child in your particular circumstances will be a big decision. It must be a labor of love."

From the beginning, Louie and Cherie were conducting their own research efforts parallel with Dr. Berg—seeking others with 7q11.23 duplication, sharing information with parents just entering into the mysterious duplication fold and learning from others who had been laboring and researching alone. Berg, who was still at Baylor, helped the Ruffinos circulate a letter to all of the geneticists in the state, informing other parents of children with 7q11.23 duplication that they were not alone—that other mothers and fathers were sharing information and ideas until the scientific world could catch up with the problem. And they were discovering interesting similarities and differences in all of the affected children they were beginning to discover, whose parents had contacted the Ruffinos to share their own stories and research. "Chloe is language delayed," says Cherie, "the opposite of Olivia who has her language developed. Then there's Jackson who has both language delay and behavioral issues."

When Cherie first met Dr. Berg, Chloe was almost three years old. Four years later she was coming along, attending first grade in a structured-learning class at a public school and beginning to speak a little. "She does not actually carry on a conversation; she gets her message delivered to you with three- and four-letter words. But she's very intelligent; she reads although her writing is poor," Cherie says.

Chloe still has a long way to go, but she has also made some significant progress. This year, five years since her diagnosis, Chloe spends part of her day in a regular second grade classroom. Although she can now communicate in full sentences, and can ask and answer questions, she doesn't always use proper sentence structure. "Instead of 'What is your name?' she'll ask "'What's name?'" explains Cherie. "Or, instead of asking 'What day is today?' Chloe might ask 'Day is?'"

Like other children with the duplication, Chloe also recently developed some behavioral issues. "She has outbursts," says Cherie. At this stage, "everything is about Chloe." In addition, she has more trouble grasping cause and effect than other children her age. "She doesn't understand that if she steps in front of a car, the car may not stop," Cherie explains. To protect Chloe from danger and help her to calm herself, the Ruffinos have placed her on a waiting list to receive a service dog.

Initially, because of Cherie's efforts, the parent network expanded to include nearly thirty families around the world—including families from Germany, Canada and Belgium. The name they initially chose for themselves reflects who they are and the mystery of why the group exists: the 7q11.23 Dup (pronounced like "doop") Group. Since that time, the Dup Group has merged with a group started by another mother who started a website at Duplicationcares.org. The other mother focuses on education and raising awareness, both among doctors and the general public. Cherie still works behind the scenes, focusing on family support. Some forty to fifty families are now involved worldwide. Although nothing can be done at this moment to help their children except to trade information and ideas, talk, commiserate and wait for researchers like Jonathan Berg to find more answers and explanations, the families have discovered some valuable basic information related to their children's previously inexplicable difficulty. Equally important is the realization that they are not alone. There is power in numbers.

CHAPTER 16:
HEALTH IN YOUR HAND

In the spring of 2007, a diabetic blogger named Amy Tenderich posted an open letter to Steve Jobs, imploring the head of Apple to create a new kind of medical machine. "I'm writing to you on behalf of millions of people who walk around wired to little tech devices," Tenderich began. "No, I'm not talking about the iPod." Diabetic people "are, of course, deeply grateful to the medical device industry for keeping us alive," she wrote, but the life saving machines tend to be terribly designed and embarrassing to wear—nothing like the sleek smartphones or media players that we all tuck into our pockets.

"This is where the world needs your help, Steve," Tenderich wrote. "If insulin pumps or continuous monitors had the form of an iPod Nano, people wouldn't have to wonder why we wear our 'pagers' to our own weddings, or puzzle over that strange bulge under our clothes. . . . [S]trangers wouldn't lecture us to turn off our 'cell phones' at the movie theater. . . . [M]edical devices are also life devices, and therefore need to feel good and look good for the patients using them 24/7."

It is people with diabetes—perhaps more than any other group of patients—who fantasize about a whole new kind of medical equipment. Their lives depend on glucose monitors and insulin pumps. Therefore, diabetes patients have started to demand, and even invent, a new class of phones that can double as medical machines. But the potential applications go way beyond diabetes. As our phones begin to keep tabs on our vital signs, they can become the portal through which all of us interact with our doctors and our health records.

Matt Tendler, a young entrepreneur, puts in fourteen-hour days trying to transform ordinary phones into cutting-edge "diabetes machines." Tendler's story starts in the fall of 2002, when he was a college freshman struggling with a mysterious ailment. Back then, Tendler would sleep sixteen hours a night and then wake up dazed, late for class. He would creep down the five flights of stairs in his dorm building, clinging to the banister. He figured he must have mono. Only weeks before, he'd been playing intramural football with the guys on his dorm floor. Now, he craved orange juice with a thirst so deep it pushed him to wander the halls of his dorm, knocking on doors. He'd plead for juice, Gatorade, even milk—anything to quench this new and terrible thirst.

The craving for liquid, for sugar, was so intense that he stopped caring whether his dorm-mates thought of him as a moocher. Juice had a magical effect on him. One sweet drink in the morning, and he would hurry off to class, feeling almost normal. And he wanted so badly to feel normal. He was pledging a frat. He was dating a girl at Tulane. If he could just sweat out this mono, he thought, life would be perfect.

February 7, 2003: Tendler remembers the date because he passed out, wound up in an emergency room in Bloomington, Indiana and finally learned what was wrong. After his diagnosis, Tendler tried to comfort himself. After all, the doctor had described type 1 diabetes as a minor annoyance. Tendler saw no reason to stop hanging out with his beer-pong-playing frat brothers.

"Remember that there are carbs in alcohol," the doctor had said—almost as if he were encouraging Tendler to indulge. And that's what Tendler did in the first weeks after his diagnosis. He partied most nights at his frat; every time he chugged a beer, he'd shoot himself up with insulin.

Now, describing that time, Tendler sounds spooked. People with type 1 diabetes call the weeks just after diagnosis and the start of insulin treatment the "honeymoon period": the body still makes some insulin on its own, and the patient can get away with behavior that would later put him in a coma. On one of those nights when Tendler glugged vodka shots, he might have dropped dead. It was only his own limping pancreas that saved him.

Five years later, Tendler had become a wheeler-dealer in an Armani suit, hurrying out the door of his West Village apartment to a finance job at a top brokerage house. He'd learned to manage his diabetes, sort of. But he hated all the crap he had to carry around: In addition to the usual cell phone and wallet, Tendler had to pack a glucose meter, a few Starbursts, an insulin pen, a pricking device, test strips. His pockets always bulged obscenely. Would diabetes force him to carry a man-purse? It seemed the final indignity, he recounted, telling his tale.

He had his eureka moment one day as he was cramming his cell phone and his glucose meter into the same pocket: the two gadgets could be merged into one. The glucose meter, of course, is the diabetic's lifeline. It tells him when his blood sugar has peaked or fallen to dangerous levels. A few bad spikes can mean death, dementia, amputation.

Over the next few days Tendler kept mulling over his idea. It wasn't just about reducing clutter, he realized. If he could plug his glucose device into his BlackBerry, he would be able to send readings to his doctor. He could load blood markers into special software; he could slice and dice his own data as if it were a stock pick, analyzing his own body until he tracked down the patterns that kept his blood sugar stable. Tendler pictured a new kind of medical device that provided everything he needed to manage his disease, from diet tips to social networks, on-call nurses and number-crunching. In short, he imagined being able to make his own blood talk to the Internet.

He was not the only person thinking along these lines. The diabetes community had been abuzz with demands for better machines—and people wondering why they couldn't plug their medical equipment into their iPod, iPhone, BlackBerry or laptop. So why didn't an "iPhone for diabetics" exist yet?

As Matt Tendler looked into the matter, he discovered the enormous legal and regulatory hurdles that stood in the way of that kind of innovation. A medical device must pass FDA approval, an expensive process that can take years. In addition, any machine that sends patient information over phone lines must comply with complicated HIPAA laws, the regulations that protect medical privacy.

Tendler's project seemed to be doomed. And if times had been different, he would probably have given up on his idea. After all, how could a twenty-four-year-old salesman transform the telecommunications industry? But these were no ordinary times. In September 2008, the stock market had shattered. Traders raced around whispering about a meltdown, financial Armageddon. Lehman Brothers—one of the titans of Wall Street—had evaporated overnight.

Tendler languished in the cold-calling room at his brokerage firm; he was supposed to work through a list of names, phoning strangers and chirping about the advantages of financial products. But what customer would entrust money to a kid on Wall Street in the midst of a crash? So Tendler began to hide out in his cubicle, mapping out a business plan for his still-imaginary company.

By this time, he had contacted Tom Xu, a programmer and engineer who had already created health apps for the iPhone that allowed patients to record and monitor carbohydrate intake, exercise, weight loss and blood pressure. Tendler and Xu figured that, from a technical standpoint, it would be easy to create a blood monitor that would plug into the iPhone and take advantage of all of its apps. One day, they even hacked an iPhone so that it would communicate with a glucose monitor. They could hold their dream machine in their hands; it worked. This machine that could change the lives of millions of diabetics would be easy to manufacture. But it was far from legal.

As far as Tendler could figure, he and Xu would need as much as $10,000 just to find out whether their machine would ever be able to comply with government regulations. They'd have to hire intellectual-property consultants and lawyers who handled FDA approval. And at the end of the process, they might learn that even though their plug-in could pass the government hurdles, the cell-phone companies still wouldn't want to partner with them. Nonetheless, Tendler could not help believing that his machine—now named Glucose Buddy—would win the day.

By December, Tendler had left Wall Street and was working on Glucose Buddy full-time out of a coffee shop called the Soy Luck Club. Because the cafe forbade cell phone calls, Tendler held his meetings out on the sidewalk of the West Village. The pharmaceutical executives on the other end of the line had no idea they were talking to a twenty-four-year-old kid who was shivering on a street corner.

Then, in March 2009, the game changed.

Apple announced that it was willing to turn the iPhone into a medical tool. At that time, Steve Jobs had his own reasons to be thinking hard about healthcare. For years, Jobs had been struggling to survive pancreatic cancer. He'd shrunk down to the size of a skeleton and was so gaunt that media pundits were gossiping about what would happen to Apple after his death.

At a media event in March, Jobs himself was absent—on leave for a liver transplant. But he was very much a presence in the room as Apple executives showed off a prototype of the iPhone that could plug into a glucose monitor and a heart monitor. Apple might now enter the medical market.

At that event, the iPhone was plugged into a glucose monitor made by Johnson & Johnson, signaling that Apple was likely to work with Big Pharma. But Tendler and Xu believed that they had something to offer that even Johnson & Johnson didn't: a community. They had already begun to develop an online community center, where diabetics could trade advice and seek help from a nurse.

For a diabetic person, maintaining good health depends on making lots of small decisions the right way, over and over again, for decades. Social support can help the patient stay on track, and so can machines that monitor the body and let the patient see results.

Of course, almost everyone faces some version of this challenge. Many healthcare watchers believe that millions of people—including nondiabetics—will eventually carry around machines that help us manage our bodies and medical records. By the year 2025, according to a RAND study, half of the American population will be suffering from a chronic disease. Half of the country will need to monitor its diets or medications. Doctors cannot be at our sides every moment. A new class of medicalized phones may help provide the services of pharmacist, coach and nutritionist. So while Matthew Tendler sees the iPhone as a potential "diabetes machine," other innovators are building apps and add-on gizmos that make it a "weight-loss machine" or a "heart-disease machine" or a "sports-training machine."

In 2009, Jen McCabe moved to San Francisco with two suitcases, a whiteboard and a plan to revolutionize the American hospital. Like Matthew Tendler, she lived with a cell phone in her hand and imagined a new kind of healthcare system, a dazzling cloud of data that a patient could tap into from anywhere. Only twenty-nine years old, McCabe had already worked in healthcare administration, drawn up policy papers and advised hospitals on how to reach patients through the Web. At twenty-five, she'd been elected to the board of directors of Medbank of Maryland.

Now McCabe wanted to do more than advise hospitals; she wanted to transform the culture of healthcare and the way we think about our bodies. And the tool for this transformation is a phone, she said in a 2009 interview. It's not just that a phone connects you to the nearest hospital; it can also connect you with your own willpower, and to the little nurse inside your own head.

One of McCabe's favorite words is "microchoice." By that she means the few seconds when you are gazing at, say, a milkshake and wrestling with yourself. In fact, even as you read the previous sentence, you might have been struggling with a microchoice. *(Milkshake? Milkshake! I could make one right now.)*

McCabe argues that we make calculations about our health all day long. On her blog, McCabe once kept track of some of the microchoices that she made in a two-hour period:

—Ate a pear and drank some kefir for breakfast. Not the French toast smothered with maple syrup . . .

—Washed breakfast down with some black tea and honey instead of coffee and Splenda.

—Made conscious effort to drink 2 whole 8-ounce glasses of water.

—Brushed teeth. Felt guilty for not flossing.

McCabe points out that she would never dare to take this list to her doctor. Physicians and hospitals aren't equipped to get involved in our daily battles with our bodies; nor do we expect doctors to help us with our microchoices. It is strange that this should be so. After all, for millions of people, it's these microchoices that spell the difference between sickness and health. After a heart attack, for instance, a patient may receive only the most rudimentary advice about transforming his own behavior. He may, for instance, leave the hospital with a few Xeroxed sheets of information about nutrition, some of which ("avoid eggs") may be incorrect.

Making good microchoices requires more than a piece of paper, or even a warning from the doctor. It requires tools and support that guide us through a constant struggle with our appetites. First, we must be prompted, nagged or cajoled into paying attention to the present moment, so that we are aware of each tiny decision. In 2008, a study by the Kaiser Permanente Center for Health Research showed that merely keeping a food diary helped people control their weight—and the more scrupulous the dieters were about recording each cookie and carrot, the more pounds they shed.

Researchers in the field of behavioral health have spent decades studying how to make people stick to diets, take their medications and avoid risky behaviors. The key, according to many studies, is to give people some way to measure their improvement. For instance a 2003 investigation began with people who had been diagnosed with type 2 diabetes; these patients had never before monitored their blood-glucose levels. The researcher gave the patients glucose meters and required them to check their levels at least six times a week. That simple activity led to an improvement in the patients' health.

To make the right microchoices we need "microfeedback." We all know that if we drink a bottle of wine every day, eventually our liver may fail, but that's not the kind of information that motivates most of us. We need to understand the implications of *this particular glass of wine, right now.*

The makers of gym equipment know this. Every exercise machine lets us measure our performance—and challenges us to improve it. Some of the information these machines provide is downright silly. Stair-climbing machines tell us how many "flights" we've conquered. Treadmills let us gloat about how many times we've run around the "track." Even so, this kind of immediate feedback is essential to our enjoyment of the exercise. It transforms a slog into a challenging game.

Imagine if we possessed a machine that turned eating, commuting to work and even sleeping into that kind of game. Loaded with the right software, a smartphone could become this kind of machine. Millions of people have downloaded iPhone apps that help them track their exercise and performance, keep a food diary or look up the calories in a McDonald's salad. McCabe believes that these games and challenges become even more powerful when we enlist the help of our friends. She invokes Weight Watchers and Alcoholics Anonymous as examples of communities that reinforce healthy habits in their members.

If McCabe had her way, that heart patient might leave the hospital with a "microchoice machine"—a phone loaded with software. The phone could connect the patient with a nutritionist, hook him up with an online mentor, help him count his calories and remind him to attend his martial-arts class. The patient might also use the phone to monitor his heart and send readings to his doctor.

For Generation Web—those who have grown up texting and Googling—it seems only natural to think of the body as an appliance that needs to be tracked, Tweeted and tweaked. McCabe tells wild tales of West Coast parties where young geeky hipsters meet to invent machines they can use to peer at the inner workings of their bodies. Some of her friends wear wires while they sleep, in order to find out how much time they spend in the REM phase—and to improve upon their performance. Startup companies like WakeMate encourage this sort of self-monitoring and measuring. Others are hacking iPhones so that the machines monitor blood pressure.

We wear machines on our bodies nearly all the time, so it's only natural that we would begin to use these machines to monitor our health. Phones connect us to other people, of course, but they also let us talk with our own blood and heart, with our urges and momentary impulses.

In October 2009, a cardiologist named Eric Topol took the stage at the TED Talks to demonstrate that the iPhone had already become a medical device. As he paced around onstage, tiny wireless monitors fed his vital signs to his phone.

He could report to the audience, moment by moment, his heart rate, fluid levels, oxygen levels and temperature.

He was demonstrating an idea, more than anything. Topol believes that an enormous amount of healthcare can happen outside of hospitals. Doctors could monitor patients from afar. As a cardiologist, he's most excited about how this technology could save the lives of heart patients; by tracking the subtle signs of a heart attack, it could detect trouble long before the patient feels a twinge.

"What you're really trying to do is preventative medicine. You're trying to detect problems before they occur, because once a big problem happens, then you're hosed," said obstetrician Cameron Powell. Powell is the coinventor of AirStrip OB, software that lets a doctor use an iPhone or BlackBerry to monitor the vital signs of a woman in labor. "If you can detect that a baby is having a hard time during labor ten minutes sooner, you can avoid problems." AirStrip OB was the first such device ever to be approved by the FDA.

Powell said that his company had to wade through red tape to win that approval, because there are so many laws that regulate sending medical information over phone lines. "[Our company] spent $12 million in a couple of years developing a security system around AirStrip." Although the promise of smartphone-based healthcare is huge, an enormous amount of regulations and laws stands in the way.

Still, that doesn't seem to discourage Amy Tenderich, the diabetes blogger who wrote the open letter to Steve Jobs. In 2009, she launched an X Prize–style competition: whoever submitted the best technology for diabetes management would win $10,000. In response, two grad students came up with the machine of her dreams: a "skin" that transforms the iPhone into an insulin-dispensing device.

The machine has a long way to go before it becomes street legal. But at least it exists.

CHAPTER 17:
ANXIETY

Back to the day when Michael Saks, the law professor and social psychologist, was waiting for the results of his blood test at the Mayo Clinic in Scottsdale, Arizona. It was holiday time, December 2009. As a Regent's Professor at ASU, a high honor at the university given to only the most important and distinguished faculty, Saks teaches just one semester a year. The fall semester, which is just ending, was his semester "off," and Saks had been living in his summer home in Flagstaff, driving down to Phoenix periodically for meetings on campus, visits with his sister, who lives in town, and other personal business, such as doctors' appointments.

Katherine Hunt, who had conducted Saks's family history weeks earlier, walked into the room. Hunt is blonde and of medium build, a plainspoken and direct person, with a lilting up-and-down affect in her voice when she speaks. She sat across from Saks at a round table, with a scattering of textbooks and binders in the shelves behind her, looked him straight in the eye and broke the news. The blood test showed that he was a carrier of the *BRCA2* genetic mutation. Saks remembers the deafening silence that followed her pronouncement. He felt jarred and numb, and momentarily went blank.

No one could have been more surprised by his reaction than Saks himself. Generally, Saks is a very calm, calculated and analytic person—a cool customer, unmoved by emotion, driven by data. But at that point in Hunt's office, he found himself uncharacteristically overwhelmed. He vaguely remembered that when his primary care doctor had first made the referral appointment it was scheduled for the breast cancer clinic. "My first thought was, 'This must be a mistake. What's this got to do with breast cancer?'" That day when he learned the results he realized it was no mistake.

Days later, after he'd had a chance to think, all of this made sense. After all, Saks was Jewish, and *BRCA1* and *BRCA2* have come to be known to some people as "Jewish breast cancer genes." Jews of Ashkenazi descent, mostly Jews from Eastern Europe, are about five times more likely than the general population to be *BRCA1* and *BRCA2* carriers. Roughly one in forty Jewish women and men of Ashkenazi descent have the mutation, and are *BRCA1* and *BRCA2* carriers. And the *BRCA* test is not simply a breast cancer test; it also means that your vulnerability to other cancers is elevated, including prostate cancer, ovarian cancer, melanoma or skin cancer and cancers of the gallbladder, bile duct and pancreas. These were complications Saks had not expected when he first resolved to do something—or at the least find out more—about his possibility of getting pancreatic cancer.

That said, Michael Saks had been vaguely aware of all this information, and much more. And the fact that he had lived his whole life with a mutant gene inside of him was not surprising. What was so stunning, however, was that it was different genetic information from what he expected.

In some ways, this is what we secretly fear when we visit our doctor's office for testing or for a complete physical. The doctor looking into a nagging cough, an ache or a pain, or just poking and probing around your body, might suddenly discover, accidentally, something entirely surprising and unexpected and horrible. When you consider all of the new diagnostic tools that are available, anyone who goes into a doctor's office for an examination these days is a sitting duck for such surprise revelations. Breast cancer, prostate cancer, heart disease, brain tumor—it's all in the realm of possibility. So you hold your breath when you enter the doctor's office—and expel a deep sigh of relief if you depart with a clean bill of health.

Each of my three friends who over the past couple years were diagnosed with pancreatic cancer went to the doctor with mild stomach symptoms— pain and discomfort, mostly—and each staggered out of the doctor's office, reeling from the news that he might have pancreatic cancer. And look what happened to Jeff Gulcher!

I told Saks about Gulcher's experience with prostate cancer; he nodded. He clearly identified with Gulcher. Which is not to say that Saks's news—having a genetic mutation—was as bad as discovering a tumor poised to spread. But generally there is something weird, discomforting and downright haunting about suddenly discovering that there's a worm, a bug, a bad seed, an enemy invader tucked away deep inside of you where it cannot be seen or heard or felt, but can nevertheless do damage to you or your offspring.

One reason genetic testing and the distribution and dissemination of genetic information have become so controversial, confusing and contentious is because such information is so personal. Genetic testing is not *about* you or your family, your career, your failings and accomplishments. It *is* you: the very essence of who and what you are. It represents the deepest of all revelations, making the most private of all of the parts of you public. Perhaps this is another reason why Saks was unable to focus when Katherine Hunt broke the news that he was a *BRCA2* carrier. Saks is a habitual note taker, but he found it nearly impossible to concentrate—let alone to write anything—as Hunt was speaking.

"I don't know where my mind went, but I had to keep bringing myself back to the meeting and writing things down to know or remember what to do next and what to be thinking about," he remembered. "My note taking was a way of staying focused. I thought I could write down everything she was saying. I would get the information down even though my brain wasn't cooperating and wanted to obsess about what the bigger meaning of it all was.

"I was trying to absorb the information in a cognitive way and assess the emotional meaning," he explained. "What is this all telling me about my future? I guess I wasn't ready to hear bad news—but, of course, are you ever ready? And how bad is the news? Nothing definite."

This is the curious thing about such revelations and information, especially about your genetic make-up. What does it mean, Saks pondered, to be a carrier of a breast cancer mutation—or any kind of mutation? That he will get breast cancer? Unlikely. That he will pass on the gene to his offspring? At sixty-three, with no children and happily married for thirty-four years, there's no real chance of that, although the information could impact his extended family. And yet the news caused a stirring inside of him.

Months later, recalling the incident, he shook his head, still somewhat surprised by his reaction. He wondered why Hunt did not divide this one meeting into two, which is the procedure most often employed by genetic counselors so that the informational and emotional needs of the patient are wholly satisfied. "It was like if somebody walked in here and told you that your new car just got smashed up by a garbage truck, but then went on to say, 'Never mind; let's keep having our conversation here and now and you can deal with the devastation of the vehicle later.' It would be difficult for you to think about anything else at that point. And that's how I felt with Katherine." Then he added: "I was able to absorb the technical and practical information, but not the emotional meaning. Those are two different things."

But the nagging idea that compounded this news and that was so unsettling to Saks at the moment was that he had consciously and systematically undergone a series of tests and procedures over the previous year, in an attempt to learn more about his risk of cancer. And now, as a result of the Myriad test, he was equipped with more information—but it wasn't the information he wanted in the first place. Now there was something else, entirely unanticipated, in the mix. It was hard not to wonder whether he had made a mistake, even getting involved in this entire genetic testing process. What had it accomplished?

CHAPTER 18:
CLIFF DIVING

Michael Saks is not a young man; he has already lived the majority of his life, at least numerically speaking. And even though he was quite taken aback by Katherine Hunt's news, he knew, down deep, that he probably would not get breast cancer. Even though the *BRCA* test was telling him that he was at a slightly elevated risk to contract breast cancer and other cancers, including pancreatic cancer, the news he received that day in December did not precipitate a crisis. He was shaken momentarily, that's all.

But for other people, more susceptible to anxiety and perhaps with more to lose, knowing too much about their possible fate can be harmful. I actually witnessed the beginning of such a scenario, as I sat in Steve Murphy's office one afternoon, observing. I say "the beginning," because a year later, the ending—if there is an ending—remains a mystery.

Arthur and Cassandra Bond were both twenty-eight years old, highly skilled professionals climbing the corporate ladder in the world of finance, both graduates of Ivy League universities. They had been married for eighteen months, and had come to Murphy's office to review their preconception testing results. Until recently, preconception testing was relatively uncommon, limited to couples who knew they might be carriers of specific, potentially harmful genetic mutations or who were attempting pregnancy later in life. Quite recently, however, many affluent couples have begun undergoing such tests as an extra precaution—and simply because additional information is available. Preconception testing was a new way Murphy was keeping his practice alive. He used the Counsyl Universal Screening Test, developed by a Silicon Valley start-up company.

Arthur and Cassandra were casually but expensively dressed; Arthur wore a blue, open-collar shirt, khaki trousers and tassel loafers, and Cassandra was in heels, a green sweater and gray skirt. She wore dangling silver ball earrings that jiggled when she laughed, and she was quite animated and chatty. Arthur was more restrained, smiling and nodding as Cassandra and Murphy conversed first about the weather and then about Murphy's growing family.

I was not the only observer in the room that day. A reporter from a local newspaper was doing a story on Steve Murphy—the Gene Sherpa—and personalized medicine, and had brought a photographer along. A graduate student studying science journalism was also present, as was an intern from a Manhattan-based medical school. Murphy appreciates a good audience and always performs well.

The reporter's story about the Bonds' interaction with Murphy was eventually published, with photographs, and used the couple's real names. I have changed the names of the couple here, but the details are as accurate as possible, considering that the Bonds have stopped communicating with me—and with Murphy.

Initially, the Bonds had not come to Murphy for preconception testing; like most people, they had not realized that preconception testing for a wide range of genetic mutations was an accessible and relatively affordable option. Cassandra had begun seeing Murphy recently for anxiety. She had been referred by Arthur's doctor (she was from out of state and did not have a regular general practice physician), who had said that Murphy was young and known to be giving patients a lot of attention as he built up his fledging practice. This was true, although part of Murphy's practice had to do with allocating more time to patients so that he could use his special knowledge about genetics to better diagnose and treat them.

Murphy adjusted Cassandra's anxiety medication and, as was his routine, took a family history. A few months later, when the couple began talking about starting a family, they realized that the anxiety medication might pose risks during pregnancy. So they visited Murphy and talked with him about preparing for children, which is when Murphy mentioned Counsyl, which would look at DNA samples to determine whether Cassandra and Arthur were carriers for any of one hundred various diseases that could potentially be passed on to their children. There are, of course, many more than one hundred ways to be carriers, but this was the limit of the Counsyl test—and it provides a substantial survey of the potential genetic pitfalls of pregnancy.

The Bonds agreed to the Counsyl test immediately. In a way, they were both information junkies; approaching new ventures with all available information at their fingertips was a way of life to them. *The Wall Street Journal* recently referred to patients like the Bonds as "patient-scientists." And certainly, patients should embrace information and keep abreast of news about ailments that affect them. But sometimes the quest for knowledge can become an obsession, and information can harm as well as help.

The test was not very complicated; the Bonds came into Murphy's office, spit into cups and that was that. Later, conferring with friends and colleagues, Cassandra learned of others who had gone through a similar testing process. One couple had discovered that they were cystic fibrosis carriers. But Cassandra wasn't worried. In most cases, both the father and the mother must be carriers of a mutation in order to pass the problem on to the baby, and, she said, "Dr. Murphy told us that based on our family histories, it was unlikely that we would have two matching carriers for any of the diseases." She was unfamiliar with genetics, but was anxious to learn more about herself and about the future health of her family.

The Counsyl test does not in any way compare to the depth and scope of genome sequencing. It examines barely a fraction of genetic material, identifying a narrow sliver of possibilities, as Murphy explained to the Bonds. He broached the subject, the results of the Counsyl test, slowly, easing the conversation in that direction. Sitting in front of Murphy's shining walnut desk, Arthur and Cassandra listened to the doctor review the results:

"Understand that a man or woman can live whole lives healthily without ever knowing about anything different in their genes," he began. "But if and when that person meets another person who has a change in the same gene"—by which he meant, a mutation—"not necessarily the same change, and they have a child, there is a risk that that child could have a whole host of problems."

Steve Murphy is well aware of the sensitivities created by genetic testing, and he was careful to present his report in an informative and reassuring manner. Murphy brought up the test results on his computer display and went through it in detail with the Bonds. He cited a list of mutations that might inhibit the processing of certain medications, followed by mutations that could cause a condition leading to iron overload. He went on in this way for five or ten minutes, all the while continuing to reassure the couple that there was little to be concerned about. Cassandra's tests indicated a slightly higher risk of a mutation in the *G6PC* gene, which elevated the danger of her not being able to properly process glycogen—sugar—but even this Murphy did not see as a problem. Cassandra was a carrier, but "with this condition, like all of the others we tested for, you need two copies to manifest." Arthur was not a *G6PC* carrier, Murphy explained. "So, not to worry," he said reassuringly.

And yet, Cassandra mused later, just listening to all of the possibilities was unsettling. "Kind of like you've just escaped a gauntlet of dangers and now you can finally take a deep breath—and thank God you are alive and not genetically flawed."

When the Bonds were ready to leave, Murphy printed out color copies of the entire report for both Arthur and Cassandra. They chatted amiably for a while about having checkups and said goodbye. It was all very casual. The meeting had taken an hour.

Later, waiting for his next patient, Murphy sat behind the shiny walnut desk in his office, joking that Arthur and Cassandra would not gloss over the detailed printout he had turned over to them. Based on their age and professions, they would immediately be poring over the graphs and charts, he predicted—they could not resist.

But Murphy was only half right. Both Cassandra and Arthur had taken time from their jobs to see the doctor, and now they needed to head to work. In fact, Arthur had said goodbye and disappeared, and Cassandra, who had stopped at home, was about to follow—she was nearly late already—but at the last minute she couldn't help going to her laptop and typing "glycogen storage disease" into Google, seeking information about her mutation. As it turns out, it was not a "ticking time bomb," to use Murphy's phrase, for their potential baby but, quite surprisingly, at least initially, for Cassandra herself.

The primary symptom of glycogen storage disease (GSD) is hypoglycemia, which, Cassandra suddenly realized, she might have. "If you look up 'hypo,' it mimics anxiety, which is why I went to Dr. Murphy initially. And then I remembered commenting when I first saw Arthur's doctor about how, when I felt anxiety, I would sometimes eat. And he said, 'Oh, you shouldn't try to get rid of the anxiety through food'—he was thinking I would become an emotional eater. But after making the connection, I began looking at it in the framework of maybe this is hypoglycemia. And the more I thought about it, the more sense it made."

Hypoglycemia, she learned, is often accompanied by seizures, information which precipitated another critical memory. "I thought back to an incident when I was middle-school age. I was home alone, and I was walking down a hallway, and I remember starting to shake, and fall down and go unconscious, and I am pretty sure I was unconscious for a few hours. When I woke up, I was really scared." She told her mother what had happened. "I thought my mom was thinking I was crazy."

But then she remembered another incident, years later. She had been out with Arthur one night, and they had had a few drinks. When they left the bar to go home Cassandra suddenly couldn't stand up, and she was shaking all over. She lost control of her bodily functions. As she scanned through articles online, putting it all together, she began to believe that she had had hypoglycemic seizures. And despite Dr. Murphy's reassurances, she began to wonder what this discovery might mean for her own future health and that of her child.

Before shutting down her laptop and leaving for work, Cassandra composed a quick and pointed e-mail message and sent it off.

Back at Murphy's office, Murphy's cell phone pinged. Murphy does not often take calls from patients, but he makes it a point to answer e-mails as quickly as possible. Murphy had been shoving handfuls of raw mixed nuts into his mouth, and washing them down with gulps out of a Mason jar of pure honey. He will nip at the nuts and honey throughout the day, aware that what you eat is as important as your genes are. Murphy took a swig from his honey jar as he read Cassandra's e-mail aloud:

"After reading through our preconception paperwork, I have a question about the glycogen storage mutation disease that I have. The paper reads that carriers generally do not experience symptoms. However I do experience what I believe are blood sugar–related symptoms and low hypoglycemia, and I had an unexplained seizure as a teenager."

Murphy responded to Cassandra's e-mail immediately, scheduling an appointment for early the following week. When Cassandra Bond returned to Steve Murphy's office, she was feeling quite anxious. Cassandra had put the issue of children on hold. She wanted the glycogen storage disease issue to be straightened out first. It had struck a chord.

There are, Murphy explained, numerous possible mutations that could lead to hypoglycemia and he couldn't really respond to Cassandra's needs without additional blood work that would map part of her genes to determine which (if any) of those mutations she might carry. Murphy then took a blood sample so that Cassandra's *G6PC* gene could be entirely sequenced in order to determine the exact variations she might have, which could explain more about her specific glycogen storage disease problems.

Cassandra and Murphy talked for more than a half hour. Cassandra left the office feeling as if she was doing the right thing, but also very much on edge, mostly because of the long wait time before Murphy would receive laboratory results. Six weeks would be a frustrating, agonizing wait—and because it was over the holidays, it turned out to be three months before she got the results.

Day by day, Cassandra became more anxious, fearing—despite Murphy's assurances to the contrary—that the blood tests would reveal terrible news. And her hunger for information—her need to know about all of the possible permutations—had actually made things worse, for she couldn't stop reading about the ramifications and side effects of hypoglycemia and glycogen storage disease. "My boss told me I should calm down, that I am suffering from what he calls 'medical student syndrome,'" she said. "You read about something which has very common symptoms, and you say, immediately, 'I have it! I have it.'"

This is the negative side of the information explosion. The Internet can help patients better understand the rationale behind the ways in which their doctors are treating them, while providing insights into the diagnosis and treatments of their difficulties and diseases. But it can also trigger nervousness and false hopes and fears. A little bit of knowledge can be frustrating and can cause anxiety attacks that are harmful and frightening, if not downright dangerous.

Most doctors have mixed feelings about their patients' online explorations. Certainly, they are delighted that their patients are well informed about their health issues and are willing to step up and take responsibility for caring for themselves. On the other hand, they fear that their patients may misinterpret the information they receive online through Google or other search engines and from direct-to-consumer testing companies.

"This whole direct-to-consumer community of empowerment has scared the shit out of me," Murphy once commented. He does not think it should be so easy to receive such potential traumatic information, especially without a qualified personal physician to guide you. Even with Murphy's counsel and support, Cassandra was upset. Imagine if she'd been alone, without any help navigating. He made a good point, of course. On the other hand, the DTCs cut into his market, which was not particularly fertile at the moment. So Murphy might have been scared by the DTCs even if they were reputable and effective.

That said, Murphy was far from alone in his resistance to DTCs. Lane Rutledge, Bruce Korf's colleague at the University of Alabama, Birmingham, observed that often the information available online, even when accurate, presents the worse-case scenario—potentially and unnecessarily upsetting family members—and can easily mislead patients into taking unnecessary and potentially harmful action. Murphy refers to this as "cliff diving."

"We recently told a mother that her baby had an 'abnormal PKU test,'" Rutledge told me. Phenylketonuria (PKU) is a metabolic genetic disorder that causes an inability to break down a specific amino acid, and that can cause brain damage if untreated. "She went online, looked up PKU test and was in the process of getting formula for PKU, as one Internet article suggested, and putting her baby on it. Well, the baby didn't have PKU." In this instance, formula would have been harmful to the baby.

While the same information available to Murphy is also available, more or less, to Cassandra Bond or other patient-scientists, Murphy's deep well of experience can make a major difference between relief and trauma, insight and confusion. It makes sense then that doctors in private practice should not only utilize their vast knowledge of science and medicine to soothe and satisfy their patients, but also to learn what their patients are reading. Instead of withholding information, doctors should become aware of the reliable information available through the Internet—and steer patients away from the information that will confuse or frightened them.

"It has been an emotional roller coaster for me," said Cassandra. "I am a person who plans for the worst. I keep trying to read everything I can to figure what this is. I know that this is not a very severe case because severe cases are found in childhood, but sometimes, as I understand it, even if you carry just one of the genes, the baby can be affected. And that usually occurs in women around my age—twenty-eight or a little older. Because, according to the literature, they start to have problems with their organs, problems with their liver and kidneys because glycogen gets stored in the organs—and can cause damage.

"I know I am dealing with a progressive disease. My only concern is what damage have I done to my organs at this point. And one of the things that can destroy your kidneys is if you have blood in your urine, and I have had a lot of urinary infections over the years. I have seen a urologist and I know I have blood in my urine—so here is another thing to worry about.

"So I am sitting here and waiting for this month and a half to end and trying not to think about it. But like I said, I am on an emotional roller coaster every day. It is hard not to think about what is on your mind day and night."

Later, I asked Steve Murphy whether he had experienced such powerfully negative reactions—and fears—from other patients, or if Cassandra's reaction was unusual. He answered with great force and frustration, almost yelling: "Lee, you have no idea. We have to be ever so careful and cautious because we are playing with fire here. People can be damaged, never get over it or live it down!"

Cassandra had promised to talk with me again when the results of her other tests were made available, and when I did not hear from her after a couple of months, I e-mailed her to remind her of her promise. She did not answer. After a couple of weeks I e-mailed again. And then again. She had given me her telephone number, and I tried that about a half dozen times over a few months, leaving voice-mail messages. Eventually, I contacted Murphy to make sure my contact information was correct. He provided Arthur's e-mail for me to try, which I did—no answer. Murphy acknowledged that he hadn't heard from the Bonds in a few months, either, and there was nothing he would feel at liberty to tell me about them. Out of courtesy to the Bonds—and respect for their privacy—I dropped the matter, with reluctance. Was it genetic information or something else that caused Cassandra to stop communicating with me and Murphy? I hope to someday find out.

There's no doubt that the power and potential meaning of genetic information is frightening and paralyzing, even to those who deal with it routinely, as professionals. I first met Michael Saks and Katherine Hunt at a personalized medicine conference, and they outlined their story and their relationship in a way similar to the way I have told it here, although not in quite as much detail as I have offered. Their photographs were on the conference website, and a video of their presentations was available online for many months. But when I asked Hunt to chat about her role as a genetic counselor and her interactions with Saks, she referred me to Mayo's vice president of Public Affairs, who agreed with Hunt that she should not discuss her work with patients, or anything else with me. After much back and forth, Saks actually wrote a letter to the VP authorizing a discussion—there was nothing to hide!—and still the VP and Hunt declined to cooperate.

There may have been many reasons why Hunt could not—or would not—speak with me about Saks or her work as a genetic counselor. But it seems to me this kind of secrecy engenders suspicion and mistrust—not particularly healthy for a field that can cause "cliff diving."

Another patient I came to know through Dr. Jim Evans—his name is Mariano Camacho—was also cliff diving, headfirst. In his case, the results of being open led to a measure of satisfaction, though not without some consternation, too.

CHAPTER 19:
DO YOU REALLY WANT TO KNOW?

As Michael Saks and Cassandra Bond could attest, people don't really know ahead of time how they will respond to genetic information about themselves and their family heritage. It's a real crapshoot, to put it bluntly. Sometimes the search for information just isn't worth the trouble; it will tell you what you do not need to know and, perhaps, what you probably should not know. And sometimes, even if genetic testing provides the answers you are seeking, it may seem like a mistake.

Very often, the information that results from genetic testing tells you nothing substantial, nothing definitive—just enough to throw you into a state of limbo. This is what happened to Mariano Camacho, a retired military special-forces petty officer who decided he needed to know whether his family—whether *he*—was cursed with the Alzheimer's gene. If there was such a gene, that is.

When Camacho made his decision to undergo genetic testing in 2009, his mother was in a nursing home, receiving nourishment from a feeding tube, totally unaware of her surroundings. Sometimes she pulled the feeding tube out and became dehydrated, Camacho told me. "Once in a while, when I get a chance to go up to see her, she recognizes me and calls me by my nickname, 'Junior.' Or she'll get me confused with my older brother—and sometimes, well, she thinks I am her husband." Two relatives, second cousins, were not in the hospital at the moment, "but," he said, "they tend to forget a lot of things now."

Camacho is fifty-six, fit and handsome with a thick head of graying hair, a neatly trimmed salt-and-pepper beard and mustache, and a high-pitched, gentle voice, slightly laced with echoes of his homeland. His family left Puerto Rico when he was thirteen and settled in Somerville, New Jersey, which Camacho has called the "most perfect" place to live. Camacho did not know his grandmother, but he has heard family stories about the ways in which memory loss and forgetfulness led to changes in her personality and eventually to dementia. His great-grandmother had suffered the same problem. His uncle, his mother's brother, had died under similar circumstances, and now his mother's older sister seemed to be in the throes of dying from dementia. "That's a lot of people in the same family," he said, "to suffer in the same way."

Dementia, by the way, is actually not a disease, according to experts at the Mayo Clinic, but a group of symptoms that might include memory loss, language difficulty or poor judgment. Alzheimer's disease accounts for 60–70% of cases of dementia, but there could be many other diseases causing dementia as well. These days, however, the word itself, "Alzheimer's," has come to symbolize the absolute worst fate to be experienced in old age. It sends a fearful shiver down the spine of anyone in their middle years or beyond who forgets too many words or faces, or experiences even the slightest evidence of short-term memory loss.

On a trip to Virginia nearly two years ago from Fort Bragg, North Carolina, where he lives, Camacho told his two daughters, Priscilla and Mercedes, that he was going to take a blood test to determine if this dementia his mother and cousins were experiencing was something that could be inherited—if it was Alzheimer's disease. Was there a gene that they were born with that would give them Alzheimer's, he wondered. Were the Camachos cursed?

He accepted the possibility that Alzheimer's was present in the family, "but until recently I personally did not give it much thought. I have been in the military all my life, and in the military you learn to take what comes at you and then you fight with all of your skill and power and determination to resist. So this was an issue not particularly on my radar screen. But I realized I had to find out for my daughters. I owed them that much."

Camacho speaks slowly and precisely; his conversation is peppered with military jargon. He frequently called me "Mr. Lee" or "Sir" until I asked him to leave out the "Mr." and the "Sir." Two yellow bracelets dangle from his right wrist: one, from Lance Armstrong's cancer foundation, says, "Live Strong," and the other proclaims, "Support the Troops." He wears a large ring with a topaz stone and an insignia he received from the Sergeants Academy after completing the two-month First Sergeants course. "I made it further than my dad," he said. "He was a staff sergeant," two grades lower in the army than a first sergeant.

"Are you frightened about what could happen to you and your kids?" I asked him.

"I have to accept reality. If that is going to be my fate, there is nothing I can do about it," he answered. "I am a strong believer that the day that we are born our book is already written for us, and if that is going to be what the Good Lord is going to give me, then—so be it. My responsibility is to inform my family."

Many in such situations share Camacho's feelings of responsibility. When a family has a disease or disability that may have genetic underpinnings, we often feel we owe our offspring (and our partners and spouses) as much information as we can provide, if the people in our family want to know.

Mercedes and Priscilla never suspected that their father would want to foresee his future in this way. This was an uncharacteristic action for a man who goes through life in a very straightforward manner. Mercedes, the eldest, 28, said. "My dad surprises me sometimes." As soon as he told his daughters what he was intending, Mercedes and Priscilla endorsed his plan. "There are some things you want to know and some things you don't, and this is one of the things I wanted to know," Mercedes said.

The memory of the last time she saw her grandmother, in 2005, haunted Mercedes; she came to New Jersey to attend her grandfather's funeral. The memory was vivid. She arrived very late: midnight. Her grandmother came downstairs, awakened by the noise. And the old woman began talking to Mercedes in Spanish and saying, "Who are you? I don't know you."

Mercedes's work schedule has not allowed time to visit her grandmother since then. But the memory and the anxiety lingered: "You know that somewhere down the line, this can be your life, and that you are witnessing it in other people, from your own grandparents. And it just flashes you forward, and you see yourself sitting there, not remembering who the people are around you who love you."

Mercedes has other health problems that may not be related to the Alzheimer's heredity. In 2004 she was diagnosed with ovarian cancer. Her ovaries were subsequently removed, and she was cancer free until 2008, when she was diagnosed with thyroid cancer. After surgery and a bombardment of chemotherapy, her disease has been in remission since 2009.

Camacho's father, Mercedes's grandfather, died from lung cancer—he was a smoker until the day he died, and although there may not be an actual cigarette-smoking gene, researchers have determined that several genes appear to dictate how likely you are to take up smoking and how easily you can quit. Researchers have also identified genetic mutations that appear to be directly linked to the number of cigarettes smokers light up daily. "My dad had emphysema and was told he needed to quit smoking," Camacho said. "I would always tell him, 'Listen to the doctors,' and he would always say back to me, 'I am strong as a bull.'"

Camacho paused for a moment to take a deep breath, thinking back to the memory and image of his father. "He was six feet tall, very athletically inclined," he recalled. "He had been a boxer, played softball, baseball, basketball, lifted weights. But when he went down, he went down like a ton of bricks. To see him lying there, the man who was as strong as a bull, in that bed, on oxygen, that to me was very devastating.

"I look at my mom now and what she is going through. This is a lady that believed more than anything in being a mother. I feel for her. Girls tend to lean toward their dads and boys toward their moms, that is the way it is in Hispanic upbringing. To me, my mom is sacred, and to see her that way, it hurts."

Camacho is not a smoker, nor are his daughters, but the fact remains that the Camachos are faced with what might be called a double whammy: cancer on one side of the family, and the "forgetting problem"—Alzheimer's—on the other.

Camacho said the word, "Alzheimer's," somewhat gingerly, as if it might bite him. He was very upset about his daughter's cancer, but it was now not the cancer—thank God, his daughter was in remission—but the "forgetting problem" that was causing him such consternation. Unlike pancreatic cancer, which destroys the victim in months, the "forgetting problem" will hang on interminably. The problem with the forgetting problem is that the victims of this disease tend to live, like Camacho's mother, in a vegetative state, perhaps much too long.

While in the Balkans, Camacho, who worked part of the year for the Department of Defense training foreign military for service in Afghanistan, had done his research. He knew it was possible to get tested for the "Alzheimer's gene," the *APOE-ε4*, discovered at Duke University nearly two decades ago. The *APOE* (apolipoprotein) gene contains instructions needed to make a protein that helps carry cholesterol into the bloodstream; a link has been discovered between a common version (or allele) of this gene, *APOE-ε4*, and an increased risk of Alzheimer's.

But Camacho also learned that even if he had the gene or genes, it is not yet possible to predict who will or will not develop Alzheimer's. Scientists are in no way certain what the link is or how the gene or genes work, exactly. And in addition to *APOE-ε4*, more than 550 genes have been studied and linked to

Alzheimer's in some way. Unfortunately, in almost all cases, researchers have been unable to replicate the evidence supporting these links.

Camacho and his daughters might be doomed—or they could have the gene, but, luckily, by some kind of miracle, escape all of the consequences.

This was not exactly what Camacho's daughters wanted to know; the little bit of information they had did not seem to go a very long way.

To complicate matters, Mariano Camacho's physician at Fort Bragg, North Carolina, had no idea that she could actually do genetic testing for Alzheimer's. She and Camacho looked it up on her computer together, and she was quite surprised. Camacho was also surprised that he knew more than his doctor about this particular test—but he appreciated her willingness to learn from a patient, let alone an enlisted man. She wrote the referral.

It was even more surprising, for Camacho, to have worked so hard to learn about Alzheimer's, waiting for months for an appointment with his primary care doctor, even going so far as to educate his primary care doctor, only to learn that the geneticist to whom he was referred, Dr. Jim Evans, at the University of North Carolina in Chapel Hill, didn't want to conduct the test.

When I asked Jim Evans why he was hesitant to test Camacho, he threw up his hands in frustration. "What good would it do?" When the *APOE-ε4* allele was first identified as a factor, the risk was estimated to be 50%. More recent estimates suggest that *APOE-ε4* might account for only 20–25% of late-onset Alzheimer's.

"My feeling all along has been that this is worthless and potentially damaging information," Evans said, "because, at this particular moment, you can't do anything to change the risk. There's no surgery, no medication, no possible cure on the near horizon, except to tell patients, to warn them, that they are, to a certain extent, in jeopardy."

It was the same old story that Michael Saks had been told, the message delivered to the vast majority of patients: Scientists know a lot more than they did a decade, a year or a month ago; research is rapidly progressing. But, in relation to Alzheimer's (or pancreatic cancer), not a lot is happening that can be taken to the bank in the near future.

"Dr. Evans spoke with a lot of candor," Camacho observed. "He was concerned, and he was doing his job, but I wanted him to realize that I was very serious and that he could not dissuade me. I wanted the test done. I came there with my mind made up. Nobody was going to talk me out of it."

"So what can you say to patients like Mr. Camacho?" Evans asked rhetorically, "to help them reconsider or to console them if the news is not good? You can bring out all of these platitudes about staying active—keeping their minds sharp and their muscles hard. But it is not going to make an impact or a difference in the end, not one bit. Even the information that we have is not robust enough—I mean, the information is not clear and concise. I might be able to tell you that you are at a twofold or threefold risk for Alzheimer's, but that really leaves an awful lot of room for uncertainty. I would feel really bad if you went to the bank and withdrew all of the money from your 401(k) and retired early based on this information, and then you got lucky and didn't get Alzheimer's at all, but now you are bankrupt, living in a cardboard box—poverty stricken."

On the one hand, Evans is being paternalistic, acting like some kind of deity guarding information from the person who, in fact, owns the information and has purposely sought it out. This sort of attitude is not uncommon in the medical profession, where patients are often treated like children, not rational or mature enough to deal with technical data and cold hard facts. And yet, the very fact that the tests are available can lead a patient to believe that there is some sort of wisdom, a magical insight that comes from a modicum of information. Knowing the risk factors—how likely you are to be victimized by Alzheimer's—can be soothing if your risk factor is low, but frightening if your risk factor is high, and somewhat misleading, either way.

The Alzheimer's mutation is not a cut-and-dried, one-way-or-the-other kind of determination. The test will tell you if you have inherited a single copy of the Alzheimer's gene and thus find yourself at an elevated risk for the disease. But you can also inherit two copies of the gene, which puts you in the "high risk" category. To complicate matters and frustrate everyone, some high-risk people may not develop Alzheimer's, while other people who learn that they don't have the gene may fall victim anyway.

"This is what I tried to tell Mr. Camacho: that the information I could provide would be of absolutely no help whatsoever—and it might be depressing and have a negative effect on himself and his daughters. What good would it do?" Evans repeated. "What good would it do?"

Most physicians, and maybe even some patients, are likely to sympathize with Evans's reluctance to test patients for the Alzheimer's gene. Knowing what might happen to you is not necessarily going to do you any good—and it could do you harm by creating anxiety.

But a study conducted between 2000 and 2003 (definitive results were published in the *New England Journal of Medicine* in 2009) portrayed another side of the story. Robert C. Green, MD, MPH, then affiliated with Boston University and currently a lecturer at Harvard Medical School's Brigham and Women's Hospital, led a team that recruited 162 adults, fifty years of age or older, who, like Mariano Camacho, had at least one parent suffering from Alzheimer's. Like Camacho, none of the subjects being studied showed outward signs of Alzheimer's. Surprisingly to the many doctors protecting their patients from potentially harmful information, the results of the study—called the REVEAL study—demonstrated that testing positive for *APOE-ε4* didn't cause lasting or significant negative effects on subjects. Green reported three major conclusions: First, quite obviously, people who learned they did not carry the gene were relieved. (In fact, there are some experts who contend that even genetic information in a positive vein—no risk of contracting diabetes, for example—can be dangerous, if it leads to false security and inflated confidence and irresponsible behavior for people who feel safe and protected.) Second, those subjects who learned the results of their tests—and the results were negative—suffered as much anxiety and depression as the control group members, who did not learn their test results. Finally, those subjects who did receive bad news were able to digest it and more or less deal with it, after a reasonable time had passed, approximately six weeks.

After reading Green's study and then having the opportunity to talk with Green himself at a meeting, Jim Evans actually changed his mind. He took a blood sample from Mariano Camacho and sent it to the lab for an *APOE-ε4* determination, on the condition that Camacho would return to Chapel Hill to receive the results in person and talk with him. Many general test results are given to patients over the phone or via e-mail or letter, and research has shown that patients are generally okay with this way of learning about their health. "I am sensitive to accusations about paternalism," says Evans, "but I continue to feel that we have an obligation to protect patients from harm or irrational acts because of the information we provide them." Four months passed from the day of the test to the day the results were shared in Evans's office.

When I spoke with Camacho a few weeks after he received the results of his Alzheimer's gene test, he seemed rather depressed and reflective—not as gung ho as he had been during our first conversation, and a little confused by the information he had been provided, and the way in which relative risk and actual risk had been presented. There's a big difference between actual risk—exactly what the risk is—and relative risk, which is . . . well, relative. A person may have, for example, double the average risk of developing, say, a certain cancer. But if the average actual risk of developing that cancer is 1 in 100, then someone with double that risk still only has a 2 in 100 chance of developing the cancer.

"They told me that I acquired the gene from both of my parents—which is not good," Camacho reported. Two parental connections increase the likelihood of developing Alzheimer's. "I am in the 95th percentile of risk for contracting Alzheimer's, but, as Dr. Evans put it, 'It's like a crapshoot. There's a 50-50 chance that you may get it and a 50-50 chance that you may not get it, even though the 95 makes it seem so elevated.' But there is no getting around the fact that I am at the high-risk end of the spectrum."

His voice grew higher, and I could hear him expel a long sigh over the thousands of miles of the telephone connection. "My father gave me a gene, and so did my mother—and other than that," he paused again and sighed, "life goes on."

"Are you sorry you asked for the information?"

"I would do it again. I am not going to stop living, and I will take life one day at a time. There is nothing else I can do."

"Did you tell your children?"

"My children weren't exactly happy when I told them. I said, 'Look, you need to know what may be coming down the pike, as they say, as you get older in life—or as I get older. You need to know that I have both genes. You need to know that this is the route that I may be going. If I do get it, you won't be surprised. You've already been told. Lord willing it won't happen, but this may be the route I may be going. Did I pass the genes on to you? I do not know."

Still, he said he didn't feel helpless, or out of control.

"I am not going to quit fighting. In the military you learn not to take things for granted or give up the fight. But I won't think about it or dwell on it. If somebody asks me, I will talk about it, but otherwise I will let it be God's will. I don't want it to occupy any of my time. And I don't want to advise other people as to what to do. I am different. I have always been told that I don't march with the same beat of the drummer—and that is very true, I don't."

The REVEAL study had been influential in swaying Jim Evans and convincing him to proceed with Camacho's testing, but as it turns out there were some limitations to the study. The REVEAL study started with 289 adult children of Alzheimer's patients, who were first contacted through self-referral or at random by telephone and deemed eligible. Those who were interested in participating had to go to a group meeting to hear the details of the study and to ask questions. Some of the participants who were initially cold-called declined to attend the group meeting, and some of the folks who came to the group meeting chose not to proceed any further. Still others opted out of the study after the blood was drawn for the test—but before the results were available. Those who went through with the study went through a one-on-one session with a genetic counselor. So at the end of the testing process, and the beginning of the analysis of results, only 167 subjects remained.

Following the disclosure of the results, they received additional one-on-one counseling. So preparation for the subjects was considerably more patient-friendly and attentive than either Saks or Camacho had received.

It is difficult to know exactly why more than half of the subjects declined to go forward, but physicians and psychologists speculated that those dropouts decided that they did not want to know "bad news." Of the 167 "survivors," three experienced psychological problems after learning the results. Green and his colleagues speculated that the adverse psychological effects were unrelated to the grim Alzheimer's news, but it is unclear how the researchers could make such a definitive statement.

In addition, there are critics, such as Sanford Gordon, PhD, and Dimitri Landa, PhD, both members of the political science department at New York University, who took issue with Green's interpretation of the data. In a follow-up letter to the *New England Journal of Medicine*, Gordon and Landa argued that the control group (who were tested but not told their results) would have been more anxious about Alzheimer's simply by virtue of taking part in the study. "From a policy perspective," the pair wrote, "one would wish to compare persons who were tested and provided results with those who were not tested at all."

Still, the results of the REVEAL study led in some interesting directions. The initial results of the study, which is ongoing, were partially amended in a follow-up analysis, conducted a year later, about how people actually responded to the information they received. More than half of the subjects in the study reported that they began to take better care of their health after they received the "bad news." They began eating differently, taking vitamins or exercising, even though they admitted that they were aware of the fact that nothing was going to help them avoid the worst if they were so affected. Mercedes Camacho reacted similarly. She immediately began reading books and magazines more often to sharpen her mind, practicing hand-eye coordination, doing word puzzles, knitting and crocheting. "I know you can't cure Alzheimer's," she said, but "they say that you can prolong it from coming. I know there's no certainty, but every little bit helps."

I asked Mercedes who "they" were, but she could not remember where or if she had read this information. Her doctors, generally, as will all doctors, recommend that patients keep busy, exercise, keep their minds sharp. Activity is good for you, and inactivity is not. But there are no reliable studies that indicate that anything can help stave off the effects of Alzheimer's—at least not yet. Mercedes, like other patients in similar situations, may feel better, psychologically, doing something instead of nothing. And on the surface, the fact that they change their behavior is a good thing, regardless of whether it affects or prevents the onset of Alzheimer's disease.

One final note: Recall that Dr. Evans agreed to provide the Alzheimer's information from the blood test only if Camacho returned to talk in person. This was a conscientious and well-meaning gesture on Evans's part, for sure; he wanted to be sure that there were no lingering questions and that Camacho would not be overly upset or feel misled. As noted, Evans told Camacho he was in the 95th percentile of risk for contracting Alzheimer's because the gene appears on both sides of his family, but that there was a 50-50 chance that he may or may not get it. Evans was distinguishing between actual risk (50-50) and relative risk (Camacho's double-genetic connection put him in the high percentile).

More than a year later, when I visited Camacho at Fort Bragg and he repeated to me that he had a 95% risk, I asked him if the numbers made sense to him. If the gene appeared on both sides of the family, leading to the 95%, then "How can it be that you only have a 50-50 chance? What does that mean?"

"I don't know," Camacho said. There was a long pause. Then we both shrugged, looked at each other, smiled and shook our heads from side to side.

CHAPTER 20:
NUMBERS

Following the results of Michael Saks's tests, Katherine Hunt scheduled appointments for him not only with a gastroenterologist, but also with an oncologist, a urologist and other specialists. "It is a funny thing," Saks reflected. "All I thought about was pancreatic cancer—but now there were all of these different doctors who were examining me and other diseases and problems to contemplate." The whole experience was so overwhelming, in fact, that he was tempted to walk away and just return to his regular monitoring routine before Mayo.

Like most professionals, Saks is busy. In addition to his classes at the ASU law school, he travels widely, meeting with attorneys and jurists interested in forensics, which is one of his specialties. He has also written a number of papers and lectures about jury deliberation. Now, in order to go through the medical process in the recommended way, he had to make time to consult with all of the specialists who would need to examine him. It was all becoming much more trouble and work than he had bargained for. He could always quit, he thought, cut the ordeal short and return to his life before genetic awareness. He would take a PSA test every year to check his prostate, and he would now do his own breast cancer examination, looking for lumps—and that would be the end of that, until something happened to him and his pancreas, or the diagnostic tools for pancreatic cancer became considerably more sophisticated. This was a tempting option.

But in the end, Saks decided to follow through on what he had started. He wasn't a quitter—and he was curious. And even though his situation turned out to be exactly as he had anticipated—pancreatic cancer was as deadly as it had always been, and there was very little going on to change that at the moment—he did have some interesting and telling realizations, especially when he reported to the Mayo gastroenterologist for his examination.

Although Saks, by taking the *BRCA* test, had entered into the world of personalized medicine, his options were not in any way "personalized," except to the extent that he had gone through the testing, the counseling with Katherine Hunt and now the series of check-ups and examinations. Basically, he had been sorted into a smaller group, separate in a way from the general population—a status that did not make a lot of difference to his overall health and his fear of pancreatic cancer or, for that matter, his treatment. Genetic medicine, at least from a diagnostic standpoint, could not yet affect him one way or the other.

"What's the next step?" Saks asked his new gastroenterologist. He didn't actually think that there really was a next step, but by this point he had committed himself to the process and was going with the flow.

"What I would like to do—what I *should* do—is to look at your pancreas and see what it looks like now, this year, and then look at it again in a year, and the next year, and the year after that and see if I can observe changes," the gastroenterologist said. That was the only way to do it—to see if something was happening to his pancreas and then to try to catch it early enough to intervene.

"But how are we going to do this?" Saks remembers his gastroenterologist putting his head back, shaking it from side to side and thinking aloud. "We don't want to subject you to too much radiation, so I think it has got to be an MRI. There is no danger of radiation in an MRI. If you get an MRI, we can get a very good look at your pancreas and we will have a starting point—a place of comparison."

Since there were no protocols, no code for such an exploratory procedure, the gastroenterologist went to Saks's insurance company and requested coverage. Saks recalled, "And they said, 'No, we won't cover it. You don't have an illness. You don't have a disease.' There was no justification for an MRI, except my family background. And that was the end of that." Neither Saks nor the doctor was surprised. So it goes for personalized medicine at this moment in time. Prevention and potentiality mean nothing, for they do not impact the immediate bottom line.

This is a major challenge confronting personalized medicine advocates. Insurance coverage will have to include potential illnesses if family histories and genetic legacies are to be taken seriously. If Saks already had pancreatic cancer, then traditional medicine—or procedures, drugs and devices developed by scientists and rooted in genetics—would be approved. Of course, if Saks already had cancer, then he would almost be dead—and no matter what his doctors tried to do his prospects for living longer than a couple of months (or at best a couple of years) would be dismal. This is the quandary the healthcare profession finds itself in: prevention—including early diagnosis and treatment—is penalized. But in order to target cancer before it actually becomes cancer and practice prevention, which is one of the primary goals of personalized medicine, insurance companies must pay for preventive testing. And for that to happen, which is the only way most patients in Saks's position could get an MRI, we would have to define and code a genetic abnormality as an illness in itself. "Even though," says Saks, "there are no symptoms."

Lee Hartwell's vision of a blood test is exactly what is needed here—a noninvasive, inexpensive way to monitor the pancreas or the liver or the heart, or whatever organ or system is imperiled. But the blood test is a long way off. And as much as Saks might wish for his insurance company to relent and pay for his tests, he realizes that this won't—and can't—happen. As a social psychologist with an interest in how law interacts with science, Saks is analytical and philosophical enough to step back and think less like a patient—even though he is the patient—and more like a policy maker, paying attention to the numbers.

"It is easier for me to think about the numbers and play with the numbers than the average patient, and fascinating to me to see that my emotional reactions didn't track with the numbers—my professional reactions," Saks told me. That is, he was initially much more emotional than he expected to be, before logic and reason, usually his stronger suits, clicked in. "How many hundreds of thousands of MRIs do we want to be paying for?" he asked.

He slipped his BlackBerry out of his pocket.

"I carry the numbers around. I carry everything I need to know—numbers, statistics—around with me, and this was something I needed to understand, to achieve some personal clarity about my potential health, so I did the research and then I did the calculations.

"In a given year," he continued, reading from his BlackBerry, "I have 78 chances in 100,000 of getting pancreatic cancer, based on current statistics. Now that is with my mutation. Without the mutation, a normal person has 13 chances in 100,000 in any given year of getting pancreatic cancer. So it goes from 13 chances in 100,000 to 78 chances in 100,000 for someone like me with my family history. So what that means," he concluded, "is that I have a relative risk of six; I am six times more likely than the average person—people without the mutation—to get pancreatic cancer."

Saks admits that the relative risk of six may sound frightening to the layperson, the guy who is not obsessed with numbers or is unaware of what the numbers mean. "I know enough about epidemiology to know that the courts get interested when they learn that a risk factor is greater than two, but think what it would mean if you took 100,000 people like me and gave each of them an MRI," he said. The advantage, from a lifesaving standpoint, is that if an MRI were given to every patient with the mutation Saks has, then doctors would discover seventy-eight cases, more or less, of pancreatic cancer starting to form. "Which means, however, that 99,922 MRIs would be money spent that didn't accomplish anything, except to say that the person doesn't have pancreatic cancer. That's the downside. And if you multiply that by $3,000—the rough cost of an MRI—and then by not only 100,000 but, say, 1,000,000 people, then that is a huge number—a vast amount of money.

"So I can understand the insurance company's side of the situation. I understand why the insurance company made that decision, and I don't know how one gets around that, unless we decide we want to spend—we are up to 17–18% of our GNP. What the heck, why don't we spend half of our GNP on healthcare and on medical tests! How does personalized medicine expect to do this?"

The answer, of course, is the hope that more inexpensive diagnostic tests will be developed to monitor and screen for pancreatic and other cancers. Two researchers, working independently, one from Johns Hopkins University and the other from the Sanger Institute in England, have discovered that pancreatic tumors are not nearly as aggressive as they were thought to be. They grow slowly, in fact, and can take as long as two decades to reveal themselves—at that point, however, the patient usually has less than two years to live and the cancer has spread to other tissues. Developing a test to detect pancreatic cancer earlier might change it from a death sentence to a treatable disease. In the current healthcare system, however, the development of diagnostics is not a high priority—though Lee Hartwell and others are trying to change this. Meanwhile, Saks and people like him remain in kind of a limbo, waiting for technology to catch up with and deal with their problems.

Meanwhile, Saks said, "I understand that we cannot be doing MRIs. Although—" and this he uttered softly with a glimmer in his eye, "it would be coincidental and helpful if one day I had a very funny pain in my abdominal area, and I went to a hospital, and they said, 'We better do an MRI to see what is going on in there.' And it turned out to be indigestion." But now, amazingly enough, his doctors would have an MRI of his pancreas! "Then at least they would have a baseline for some future comparison."

This may sound like an unlikely scheme, but Saks has mentioned it to me a couple of times, and I am fairly sure that if his anxiety were ever to substantially increase, he might just suddenly come down with a severe case of indigestion that might well lead to an MRI. I think I would do that, as would many people I know. And physicians are often cooperative because the information can be helpful, if not downright necessary, and protect them from litigation and ease a patient's anxiety. Manipulating the system is not unheard of; doctors do it to skirt rigid regulations, in order to better understand and diagnose their patients.

"So that is one interesting thing to think about," said Saks in a very conspiratorial tone. "And here is a second interesting thing." He paused and nearly whispered, as he shook his head, saying, "You don't hear me worrying about my prostate!" There's a big difference, he said between a cognitive reaction to disease and the specter of death, and an emotional reaction.

What he learned, said Saks, is that even with an increased risk of six, his chances of getting pancreatic cancer were pretty slim. Here he had more numbers to share from his BlackBerry: "In any given year, I had an eighth of one hundredth of one percent of a chance of getting pancreatic cancer, but now with my *BRCA*, I have a 32% probability—or to put it another way, one chance in three—of getting prostate cancer. Not an eighth of a hundredth of one percent, but a 32% possibility by age eighty." Admittedly, most prostate cancers won't kill him—he will probably die before they become life threatening. The urologist with whom he also met at Mayo explained that there were different strains of prostate cancer—and the probability of getting the dangerous strain was only 5%. Yet, calculating the numbers again, "I have a fifty-eight-times-greater risk—I am fifty-eight-times more likely to die from prostate cancer than from pancreatic cancer.

"So, rationally—by the numbers—I should be living in terror of prostate cancer. But I still can't get emotionally involved. It is still the pancreas that worries me. And I am sure it is just because of the horror of watching what pancreatic cancer did to my mother. So this is my point—the emotional and the cognitive don't match up in situations like this.

"I teach at the law school but I am a psychologist, and psychologists are interested in cognition and emotion, so it is actually very interesting to watch myself take in cognitive information and see that the emotional responses are not correlated properly with the information. I think that that goes on a lot in many societal decisions. Human beings are not great decision makers in many ways because our emotions drive our decisions more than our cognitions in many areas. And this is one of those areas. I mean, suppose somebody said, 'We have a new monitoring test and we can only give you one of them—one that will monitor for pancreas and the other for prostate.' Now I should say prostate, but I think I would irrationally choose the other one: pancreas.

"It is all probability and odds—and that is something that I think about professionally all the time. What do you do with probability? In deciding whether a person should be executed or sentenced to life in prison, one of the factors to be taken into consideration is the probability of future dangerousness. What does it mean to say that someone has the probability of future serious dangerousness? How do you translate probabilities into decisions? This is all kind of the mystery that I have worried about professionally.

"It is easy to do when you are talking about large populations. We can think about the cost effectiveness. Useful stuff. But when you turn it into an individual, it is very hard to make choices using probabilistic information. And epidemiologists and doctors like to think in terms of relative risk, and courts also like to think of relative risk, as do public-health people. We can save only so many people in the population—we make cost/benefits decisions."

Later, Saks was in touch again about his odds of getting prostate cancer. He explained that he'd made a miscalculation: "I was mistakenly comparing the annual risk of contracting pancreatic cancer to the lifetime risk of contracting high-grade prostate cancer." After checking the National Cancer Institute's SEER website, Saks learned that the annual mortality rate from prostate cancer is 24 per 100,000. "For pancreatic cancer, since 98% of those who get it die from it, we can say the comparable rate is 76 per 100,000 per year. That means the risk of my dying of pancreatic cancer is three times that of dying of prostate cancer. So my whole line of thinking there was wrong," he explained.

Saks was, of course, relieved to discover that his risk of dying from prostate cancer was so much lower than he had originally thought. But he was also glad to learn that, ironically, his emotional response may have been on target after all. "I'm pleased to have my feelings and the data come into harmony," he said. Nonetheless, his experience illustrates how patients—real people with health problems—don't think so analytically when they are imperiled. The human brain doesn't work with numbers so well, especially when the numbers affect them or those they love. "We are storytellers," Saks said. "We are not meter readers by our genetic inheritance. We sat around campfires telling stories to our fellow cavemen. They didn't sit there with their calculator watching the fire and counting things."

Even for a man as analytical and academic as Saks, when the situation becomes very personal, statistics can be minimized or totally forgotten.

"The cancer I really should be scared of doesn't make me anxious," he said, before realizing his error. "Is it because there are interventions for prostate cancer and not pancreatic cancer? No, the truth is that I am reacting in a totally irrational manner. It is like people who are afraid of flying, but are not afraid of driving. The odds of getting killed in a traffic accident are vastly greater than the odds of getting killed in an airline accident. But for some reason, the numbers don't carry the emotional weight that they should."

I recently asked Michael Saks if he is now giving himself regular breast cancer examinations, as he has been repeatedly advised.

"I should. I am supposed to do it the first of every month, but I am bad at doing that."

"Maybe because you don't want to know?"

"No, just too busy. I am getting ready for work today, so I say to myself, 'Maybe I can do it this weekend.' It is just procrastination. If they said that there was a test for pancreatic cancer, a self-exam, and if I were not doing that then I would think that I am avoiding it. But really, if there were such a test, I would do it every day." He added, after pausing to think about what he said: "It is true to say that pancreatic cancer is horrifying and that that horror has been imprinted on me and I am imprinted on that disease. But there's a lot of disconnect between factual knowledge and emotional knowledge. That is one thing I have learned from this experience. The other thing I have learned is that there's quite a lot to worry about, if you are inclined to worry. But now I have a different attitude. The fear is with me and will always be with me, but it is less pressing."

CHAPTER 21:
INNOCENT VICTIMS

And so, Michael Saks has traveled the personalized medicine path as far as science to this point allows. He has pushed the limits of possibilities open to the average knowledgeable patient, or at the least to those with good health insurance. In an effort to understand and come to grips with his genetic inheritance, he has changed doctors in order to be affiliated with a more genomic-sensitive institution. At that institution, he has given a thorough family history to a qualified genetic counselor, consulted with relevant specialists in response to the results of his *BRCA* test and made a commitment to regular examinations and family history updates.

So was it now time to stop focusing so much on his biology and his fear of pancreatic cancer and get back to living his life? Not quite. The discovery of information about your genetic make-up and what might happen to you because of it brings forth an added responsibility. Do you inform your relatives of the risks that you all share and, if so, *how* do you inform your relatives? And where do you draw the line?

On that surprisingly difficult and nerve-wracking day when Saks met with Katherine Hunt, his genetic counselor, to review his *BRCA* test results, Hunt had informed him that it was considered good practice—the appropriate thing to do—for patients to inform relatives of any elevated genetic risks, not only for pancreatic cancer, but also for prostate and breast cancer and all of the other potential red flags that the *BRCA* test revealed. This made sense to Saks. It was obviously his responsibility, or at least it could be interpreted in that way. So he sat down, drafted a letter and sent it to Hunt to fact-check. He then mailed letters, along with copies of the official Myriad *BRCA* test results, to his brother, sister and first cousins on both sides of the family, as it was unclear which side of the family was the carrier.

Thinking over his actions, it occurred to him that some of his relatives could be upset to learn that they had a cousin or sibling at elevated risk for so many dangerous possibilities, but he figured that they were already aware that family members had died from cancer, so in a way, he thought, "I wasn't telling them something they shouldn't already have known."

Some time later, Saks happened to mention his involvement in the personalized medicine process to Gary Marchant, a colleague in ASU's law school. ASU's involvement in personalized medicine extends throughout the campus, from nanotechnology to biodesign and law. Marchant invited Saks and Hunt to meet with a class of students involved in the Genetics and Law program, which he directs. They accepted.

That day, Saks told his story about his pancreatic cancer heredity and the circumstances under which he had come to meet Katherine Hunt and give a detailed family history—and finally how and why he had reached out to his family.

After Saks and Hunt described their interactions to the group, during the Q and A session a few of the students questioned Saks's actions regarding his relatives. Should Saks have sought informed consent from his relatives before sending the information, they asked. What made him think that his relatives were interested in learning about their biology and their potential fate? What if, in fact, they didn't want to know? "You may well just be dumping on them," one of the students stated. "Maybe they didn't want to know the risk—and maybe they would be unable to deal with the worry of it all. Maybe this wasn't a particularly good moment in time to burden them?"

This line of questioning came as a surprise to Saks. Until that moment, he had not given much thought to the ramifications of his family letters; he had sent them because Hunt had suggested it, which, he knew, she had been ethically bound to do. But the students made a good point. Although Saks himself wanted to know more about his genetic inheritance, even he had been somewhat overwhelmed by the information he received, even with Hunt sitting by his side, explaining the results to him. What might his relatives think, and what sort of reaction did his letters precipitate? Theoretically, the information may have been helpful, but in no way could his news be considered "good." "Did you ever consider writing them and asking them if they wanted you to share that information?" the students asked him. "If they did, you would send it—and if not, you could keep it to yourself."

The idea of surveying his relatives before sharing information with them appealed to Saks, at least initially, but then as he thought further he wondered, "What would the first letter say? In fact, the moment you say anything to them about genetic testing, you are signaling that there's some bad news to be learned, and right then and there you are creating anxiety. You wouldn't ask them, otherwise. They are probably going to be more fearful by asking them in advance, than if they get the real information, directly." On the surface, this sounds rather silly, but it isn't. Information, no matter how potentially helpful, can be dangerous and harmful. Mariano Camacho had been able to process and deal with the information he had received—at least so far—but Cassandra Bond had not done so well.

In the end, Saks's letters elicited little by way of response. Only two recipients responded relatively quickly, and in both cases briefly, with polite acknowledgments. "But I got no real bad reaction—no negativity and no anger, although I don't know if silence is an alternative to anger in this case, or if the silence is just . . . silence," said Saks. "We are not a deeply communicative family. We see each other if we happen to be in the same place at the same time, but we're not in regular contact."

As a legal scholar, Gary Marchant predicts that there will soon be a floodgate of legal issues to confront as the personalized medicine movement gains traction. Sometime soon, lawyers will recognize that the convoluted connections among friends, relatives, spouses and their doctors and healthcare providers will need to be untangled and defined and debated in court.

At this particular time, said Marchant, patients get off scot-free, legally. Patients may have self-imposed moral or ethical responsibilities to fulfill, but there are few legal precedents. "There's a case in New York of two daughters whose mother died of breast cancer," said Marchant. The mother had remarried and the stepfather, because he was the legal spouse, had access to his wife's medical records. Because of animosity between the stepfather and the two daughters over the estate, the stepfather withheld his wife's medical records from her children. And since they knew that she had died from breast cancer, they sued for access—one of the rare cases you see of patients suing people for genomic information.

A similar case in South Carolina involved a husband and wife in a custody dispute. One of the wife's parents had Huntington's disease, so there was a 50% risk that the wife would also fall victim to Huntington's. The husband asked—

and the court subsequently ordered—that as a condition of getting custody the mother had to get tested for Huntington's. The husband's actions might be described as mean-spirited, but it was also relevant information for a judge to take into consideration before awarding custody.

Genomic information might also one day become relevant in relation to whether a man and woman ever become husband and wife. Most people, now, consider whether they are emotionally and physically—and perhaps also economically and culturally—compatible. But now a new evaluative measure may become more crucial in partnering—that is, are the men and women genetically compatible? Someday, perhaps not too far in the future, couples might undergo testing like the Counsyl preconception test the Bonds took, even before deciding whether to marry.

For now, situations of patients suing patients are rare, although not surprisingly there has recently been an increase in the number of patients who are suing doctors for sharing and/or withholding genetic information. So far, these suits have generated more confusion than precedent. Marchant cited two cases, one from Florida and another in New Jersey. Both cases involved children of parents who died of hereditary diseases. Now the children were suffering from the same diseases, and were suing their parents' doctors for not sharing the information—for not warning them of their own vulnerability.

"In both cases," said Marchant, "the court ruled that there was a duty of the doctor to have the information passed on to other people at risk in the family." In other words, both courts agreed—so somewhat of a precedent was established. The courts disagreed, however, on the process the doctors had to follow to fulfill their responsibilities: "In the New Jersey case, they said you fulfill that duty by telling the patient to tell their family members, and then you have no further duty. But in Florida, the court said you actually have a duty, if the patient isn't going to tell the family members, to go around the patient," Marchant explained. That is, in Florida, the doctor is duty-bound not to heed the patient's objections, to go around the patient if necessary, in order to make certain family members receive the information.

Even in the absence of clearly defined legal obligations, these kinds of dilemmas are extremely fraught for doctors, because it is nearly impossible to predict what patients want or how they will react to news. Marchant referred to a published paper he had read recently, written by a doctor faced with such a dilemma. A woman—the doctor's patient—took a *BRCA1* test and visited the doctor's office, accompanied by her spouse and children, to review the results. First the doctor brought the woman, the mother, into his office for a private conversation, during which he broke the news that she had tested positive for *BRCA1*. He explained the risk to the woman and urged her to inform her eighteen-year-old daughter, who was sitting in the waiting room waiting for her mother, and to suggest—urge—that the girl be tested, too. Then, the doctor accompanied the woman out into the waiting area and watched as the mother smiled and exclaimed: "It's great, everybody. Not to worry. I tested negative. I don't have the breast cancer gene!"

In the article, the doctor wondered how he might have responded. The woman was misrepresenting the message he had communicated to her—right in front of him. She was lying to her daughter, obviously so that her daughter and the rest of the family would not be burdened with worry. But now the daughter's got a false reassurance. She knows there's a family history of breast cancer, but she assumes that because her mother doesn't have the gene, she's probably also free and clear and won't ever think about getting tested.

"You get these weird scenarios popping up all the time," said Marchant, "and it's very cloudy," from both legal and ethical points of view. If you are a doctor, think of the challenges, Marchant continued: Do you go around the patient and report directly to the relatives, if you feel they have a right to know? But then, how do you find out who all the relatives are? You don't get a list of names and addresses of all of a patient's relatives. And then what happens if they sue you because you have provided information that upset them, information they did not know existed and did not want? You have frightened me, they might contend—I have a right not to know!

The silence from Michael Saks' relatives lasted for close to a year before he received a third response, from a cousin who wrote to tell him how much she appreciated the fact that he had reached out to her. "She told me she was going to get tests—and her concern was for the breast cancer. That is what her mother died of."

Although he was comfortable with his actions, Saks recognized the inherent complications. Although we call it personalized medicine, how personal is personal, he wondered. The actual personalization can travel a long way and involve many players. It entails a network of not just doctors and patients, but of relatives who may bring in other relatives, not necessarily from the same side of the family. We are all connected by our genetic heritage, in one way or the other—so how or when does our responsibility end?

Legally, said Saks, Katherine Hunt owes no duty to a person who is not her patient. If a doctor is walking down the street and sees somebody lying in the gutter who needs medical care and he walks on by, he has no responsibility or liability because the man on the street is not his patient. If the doctor does treat the man lying on the street and then sends the patient a bill for services, the patient will have to pay the bill, even if he was unconscious while being treated.

"What if, on the other hand, my employer sends me to a doctor for a physical because he is thinking about promoting me to vice president and wants to see if I am fit and healthy and the doctor reports that I have early-stage cancer? The doctor tells the employer—not the patient—for that is whom he has contracted with. The employer decides not to promote me based on this information— after all, I am not going to be around much longer—and eventually I get the cancer. And when I find out that the doctor knew in advance my prognosis and did not tell me, I sue him. So, what happens?

"I won't win. The courts have held that the doctor owed me no duty. Maybe an ethical duty, but not a legal duty. So Katherine or the doctor are off the hook."

But what are the ramifications of keeping information to yourself in Michael Saks's particular situation? Or for the Camacho family? After all, by sharing information with your family, you are also trusting your family with information about your own life and fate—and perhaps making yourself vulnerable in the process. With whom will your relatives share the information you have shared with them?

"There are so many different permutations of what could happen by sharing or withholding this information and what the reactions would be if you do tell them and if you don't tell them," said Saks. "Suddenly I have information that is not only relevant to me but also to them and I can tell them or not tell them. They can be angry to have it shared, or angry to not have it shared. This could mean so much. It might have been their last possible chance to avoid dying, to take steps to avoid disease or prolong life. In a way it is not personalized medicine. I can't use the word 'socialized' because that means something very different in this day and age, but in a way it does involve a huge network of things touching on family, science and business."

Perhaps, Saks suggested, this approach to medicine is "universalized." By this, he meant that with the advent of personalized medicine the whole idea of privacy and private information has become turned around. Already, with Google and other search engines and social networking sites like Facebook and LinkedIn, we no longer have a hidden past. James Frey, the author of the "memoir" *A Million Little Pieces*, who made up many stories and details in his book, learned this when the website The Smoking Gun decided to fact-check him, as did former congressman Anthony Weiner, who partially exposed his private parts on Twitter. Today, Americans live in public; privacy is now only an idea—not a reality. For most of us, there's a cost-benefit analysis involved in much of this: do you, for example, sign up for the grocery card that saves you money on gas but tracks your every purchase, allowing your grocery store to market directly to you more effectively than ever before? Some people might decide not to share their data; most of us, however, it seems, go along. It's just information about what kind of bread we've bought, right? Relatively insignificant.

For people who are sick and perhaps dying, however, the stakes are obviously much higher: they can no longer expect to suffer in silence and at the same time discover new ways to survive.

If you investigate PatientsLikeMe, the site started by Jamie Heywood in order to save his brother's life, you'll find yourself in what seems like an alternate universe, one where people feel comfortable revealing the kind of intimacies that they would hold back anywhere else. Each member of the site creates a profile that doubles as a medical record. There, they log symptoms such as depression, constipation and excess saliva. It's possible to click into the life of a patient and find out what drugs she took yesterday, how many hours she slept and how gloomy she felt. Most of the members also opt to tell a story about themselves. These short autobiographies offer gut-wrenching glimpses into private battles with illness.

For instance, one patient in the "epilepsy community" explains the onset of his illness this way: "I was on the job taking the written test to renew my license to drive an eighteen-wheeler . . . when I had my first grand mal. That was thirty years ago and I have not been able to drive since. I have now had four brain surgeries . . . In spite of all that I still work and have been a federal employee almost thirty-three years."

Another member gives a concise history of his spiral into depression: "I was brought up by a prison-guard father so it felt like I did time in prison most of my life. I turned to booze and drugs to cope."

Of course, the members of the site can choose a privacy setting that will allow them to hide their profile from all but trusted friends. Still, thousands of people opt to share their profile with everyone—even those who are merely lurking on the site. It's hard not to be touched by this openness as you click through the profiles on PatientsLikeMe; all these people have chosen to trust in strangers, offering up their carefully collected data to help others, in hopes, of course, that pooling everyone's knowledge might lead to a cure.

Jamie Heywood takes this as the natural order of things. He believes that PatientsLikeMe has attracted thousands of active members because most people would rather share information than horde it. "Privacy is a selfish act," he fulminated. "Privacy is a fundamentally anti-social, selfish act, and it is harmful." We all, he said, have an innate need to trust each other and form communities. "We serve our families. We serve our friends. We serve our colleagues. We work together to collaborate on everything. So the concept of privacy is almost a rejection of the fundamental component of being human, which is collective action . . . I think in the end, openness produces a much healthier society."

Of course, Heywood is correct, but he is being overly idealistic and impractical in an era when scientists, doctors and even patients themselves are hogtied by red tape and fears of litigation. Consider this conundrum: Gholson Lyon, a research scientist at the Children's Hospital of Philadelphia's Center for Applied Genomics, and the director of neuropsychiatric genetics at the Utah Foundation for Biomedical Research, learned that one of the women in a family he had been studying over an extended period was four months pregnant. She was going to have a boy—and this was an immediate red flag to Lyon because during the course of his research he had discovered that some of the boys in the family were born with a constellation of very similar and telling symptoms. These boys died of cardiac disease before their first birthday, and Lyon was convinced that a genetic mutation was causing the disease. The most prominent symptom— thick, wrinkled skin—was the clue.

So what to do about the woman who was four months pregnant with the boy? The answer would seem quite obvious: Lyon should inform her immediately, so she and her family could make an informed decision as to the best way to proceed.

Obvious, perhaps—but for Lyon, not possible. Federal law prevents researchers from sharing information related to genetic mutations with patients and their families—until and unless results are confirmed by a certified clinical laboratory. Because of the extra time and expense, most researchers, thus far, have not made it a practice to go to certified laboratories. But now, because of this law, a number of researchers, recognizing the possibility of ending up in a position like Lyon's, are beginning to routinely do their studies using certified laboratories when possible.

This is an important development. More and more people are enrolling in studies in which their genomes are being sequenced—5,000 more or less in 2011, a number that will quintuple by the end of 2012. The results, if indeed an uncertified laboratory did the processing, will not be available to participants of studies until the research is published, which could be two or three years after the sequencing has taken place—if ever.

Yet, timing is often of the essence, and such information can make a big difference to patients and families, as a pediatric geneticist from the Medical College of Wisconsin in Milwaukee recently demonstrated. David Dimmock and his colleagues sequenced the genome of a baby with acute liver failure, discovering in the process two mutations in a gene ironically named "Twinkle"— ironic because the gene causes neurological and eye diseases, as well as liver disease.

Normally acute liver failure leads to liver transplantation, even for infants. But in Dimmock's experience, the presence of the mutation negated the transplant option. He recommended against it, the transplant was not performed and the little girl died when she was six months old. "This was not a happy ending," Dimmock admitted, but then added, "but in a sense it was." The child was spared from the pain and suffering of the grueling surgery, which would have extended her life by only a few months, if that. If Dimmock had not used a certified lab, he would not have been able to recommend that the girl's parents opt out of surgery, because, like Lyon, he would have been prohibited from sharing the child's genome sequencing results.

There was no happy ending for Lyon's patient, however, in any sense of the word, although there was a bit of irony. The baby was born, as Lyon knew he would be, with the disease, which is called Ogden syndrome. And the week that Lyon's paper discussing the mutation was published was the week the boy died.

The truth is, there are many levels and degrees of privacy—one for the sick and one for the healthy, one for scientists and another for physicians. But if you've ever had a major illness, you know that you want the most thorough treatment, with all of the sensible and available options. You know and have probably come to accept that other people—nurses, doctors, technicians—will probe your naked body, cut into your flesh, piece together your secret history, examine your stool samples and ask your spouse about your urination habits, among other things. Repeatedly. And almost all people who are very ill or who have loved ones who are ill would trade in their privacy, without an instant of regret, in order for themselves or their loved ones to be restored to health.

CHAPTER 22:
GOING BACK TO THE FUTURE

I have been in touch with Steve Murphy on a regular basis from the time I first met him in 2007 until now, and I have visited with him quite often. Through these years, he has experienced many ups and downs—actually, mostly downs—until quite recently. I give him credit, a young man trying to play at a level that might have been above him, forced into debt but hanging in and surviving—and then some. Whether his idea for a successful personalized medicine practice on Park Avenue was ill advised—or whether the vision of a personalized medicine private practice, anywhere, is ill advised, at least at the moment—is hard to know right now. Certainly, the crashing economy during the years in which he was struggling to get started was an impediment. But even if the economy had been healthier, and even if Murphy had networked and promoted his practice more successfully (an unlikely scenario given his age, lack of experience, contacts and funding), the odds were still against him.

Finances were only one issue. Murphy took on too many responsibilities too quickly, as young and ambitious men and women are often guilty of doing. The demands of his many masters eventually got the better of him, especially after his wife became pregnant for the second time; a few things had to go, beginning with his genetics fellowship at Yale. Commuting from Greenwich to Park Avenue to New Haven almost every day to see patients and conduct research was simply too much. And then there was the annoyance and frustration of working in those "ivy-covered towers" he had complained about—where the academy had very little connection to the real world. Some of his colleagues in the laboratory hadn't seen a patient in years. This was not the kind of medicine he had envisioned practicing, as a student.

In 2009, after coming to the conclusion that his idea of an exclusive personalized medicine practice was either impractical or simply ahead of its time—or both—Murphy returned to Greenwich and started a private practice in general medicine, just like many of his colleagues in the town. He had finally realized what he was not doing, and what he needed to do. In his general practice, he began treating *his* patients—not referrals, but those who came to see him directly. They did not come to him because he was a personalized medicine proponent; they came because he was new in practice, was looking for patients and would see them right away and give them concentrated time and attention. They stayed with him because of his first-rate and friendly bedside manner and his willingness to spend time listening to patients' stories, no matter how long it took them to spin their tales of sickness, loneliness, suffering, family ailments . . . whatever they needed to talk about that was affecting their health.

I think back to the time in 2007 when we met my friend on the street near Murphy's Park Avenue office and my friend mistakenly assumed that personalized medicine meant what the words said—that doctors could be friendly, more personal, more attentive and responsive to patients. And I recall that Daniel Von Hoff at TGen said the same thing to me, which was why he had told me the long and circuitous story about the patient walking to Kentucky Fried Chicken in his new Adidas shoes.

Personalization begins with listening. Listening is the key to diagnosis, and the beginning of treatment.

Murphy's discovery was that personalized medicine had to start there, with listening to patients and gaining their trust. Then he could build up to genetics and high-tech tools. With this change in Murphy's circumstances came a change in his persona—the way he branded himself, his spin, so to speak. Now, he was no longer the first private practice personalized medicine physician; he was just a guy, a doctor, who thought a lot more about genetics than most of his colleagues and competitors did. He also used the basic genetic tools more, and took advantage of cutting-edge technology whenever possible.

"It comes down to personalization, real personalization," Murphy told me. "Knowing someone's Plavix metabolizer status by heart and knowing their child's birthday at the same time. Understanding who that person is—which will bring them back for more visits and generate word of mouth. It really does begin with family history, which opens up an ability to talk about things that doctors don't often talk about—things that matter the most—which leads to better medicine and back to genetics in the long run, and helps you to get better response from the patient and a better buy-in. You begin with the basics," Murphy insisted. "This is only logical."

* * *

Steve Murphy and Lee Hartwell are not acquainted, but they would certainly agree about beginning with basics—although what Murphy, as a doctor, means by "basics" is somewhat different from Hartwell's definition as a scientist. When Hartwell talks about "basics" today, he means diagnostics—recognizing diseases and doing something about them before they cause insurmountable problems for patients.

Hartwell was nearly sixty-two years old when he was presented with the Nobel Prize, an esteemed scientist who had achieved the most prestigious award and position possible in science. It might have been the perfect time to retire, you might think, and to ride his bike more. Or, he could have continued to work in the laboratory and lead the Fred Hutchinson Cancer Research Center. But Hartwell had actually taken the job at the Hutch as a learning experience to fill a gap in his own knowledge bank; he knew that a lot of the basic fundamentals he had established were important to treating cancer, generally, but he had begun to realize that he did not understand how his work in the laboratory played out in the clinic, the real world of sickness, life and death, which Steve Murphy and many other doctors knew so intimately. Hartwell did not have an MD, after all.

At the Hutch, Hartwell confirmed something he had long suspected: that there was an unfortunate disconnect between the way scientists work— beginning with the basics, gathering all available information about the subject matter they were studying and then analyzing and using the information to further their efforts in the laboratory—and the actual practice of medicine in the real world.

Scientists, Hartwell realized, had the best measurements possible at their fingertips, and more information than ever before, but despite the available technology, the incredibly powerful computational forces at our command, "We don't have very good measurements of people's health . . . We don't have very good measurements of disease," Hartwell concluded. This didn't make sense. It was illogical.

"The approval of new drugs by the FDA is around thirty or so per year," he told me one day during a conversation. By drugs, he meant medications that treat or cure disease.

Then he posed a question: "But how many new diagnostics go through the pipeline?" A diagnostic—for example, Oncotype DX for breast cancer—

provides an indication of whether a patient has a certain disease and sometimes can also provide information as to how the patient might respond to treatment.

I didn't know the answer to Hartwell's question, so he answered it himself: "Less than one."

"Are you serious?" I responded. "Less than one a year?"

"I am perfectly serious," he replied. Scientists are helping to create therapies, drugs, but they do it, Hartwell said, "blindly," often with very little understanding of the disease they are attempting to treat and cure. Better understanding can lead not only to better treatment, but also, and more importantly, to earlier detection. The goal, obviously, is to detect disease at its earliest stage so that we can intervene before it progresses to a point where it is hard to cure.

Cancer is a prime example. When cancer is detected early, before it starts to spread, it can generally be removed by surgery. Over 90% of cancer patients, said Hartwell, can be cured at this stage, whereas if the disease has been left to a late stage, after the cancer has left its local environment and spread throughout the body, then patients are very rarely cured. This same pattern, more or less, applies to all diseases. If diabetes, for example, is detected early, patients can maintain a healthy lifestyle. But if left unchecked, diabetes can cause complications such as kidney failure, loss of limbs and all kinds of other debilitating effects.

But according to Hartwell, "Diagnostics cannot get funded in the United States. The reason is because there is little financial return for it. Diagnostics just don't pay a billion dollars like a drug."

Essentially, most drugs that make it to market are developed either in the laboratories of nonprofit research facilities (mostly university medical centers) or in the private sector, such as in pharmaceutical companies. At some point, the drugs are tested on patients, in clinical trials. There are many decision points in drug development, especially as it becomes clear what the drug will do and how many people it will help, and in almost all instances, the pharmaceutical companies are the gatekeepers; since they finance drug development and marketing, they choose which drugs to invest in. But the researcher—the scientist—comes before the drug company, and here is where the beginning of the breakdown occurs. If the scientist cannot raise money for research into diagnostics, then the scientist will pursue other avenues. And because, says Hartwell, diagnostics are not "sexy, not cutting edge" and perhaps not profitable, there are few funds made available for diagnostic development. Why is there no money for the development of diagnostics? A partial answer is the agency with a $30 billion research budget to parcel out: the NIH.

In 2011, Hartwell and the Center for Sustainable Health forged a number of agreements with medical centers in Taiwan and China. He is optimistic that medical centers in India will soon be added to that list. He hopes to work with medical centers whose leaders have the understanding, patience and resources to do the research necessary to develop effective diagnostics.

"The people most receptive to the idea of diagnostics," Hartwell said, "are those responsible for national healthcare systems and frightened by the rapidly rising costs of affordable healthcare—costs are going through the sky."

But wasn't it quite clear, through the Obama healthcare plan and the continued debate in Congress, that we in the United States are worried to death about containing healthcare costs and that we are pledged to do something about this problem?

"They talk about it, but nobody is really responsible in the United States for containing healthcare costs. It is going to cripple the country," Hartwell emphasized. "It is the biggest threat to the national budget."

The government must have resources to address this problem. The government's money is allocated to the NIH for research, however, and so, because diagnostics are not high on the NIH agenda, there has been little progress made in this area. Hartwell explained that this process works differently in other countries. In Britain, for example, research is funded from two different agencies. The MRC—the Medical Research Council—is like NIH and funds exciting new breakthrough basic science. But there are other funds in the National Health Service, which go toward applied research for healthcare dedicated to outcomes and controlling costs. "We don't have that."

On the one hand, looking at the healthcare system in England and the way in which healthcare there is rationed, I was happy enough to trust the NIH—and to not want the United States to adopt a socialized medicine system. But I was surprised to hear Hartwell speaking out so adamantly, on the record.

In most cases, scientists at universities reliant on research funding, and the universities generally, are reluctant to publicly criticize the hands that feed them, especially the NIH, where the pot is so large. But Hartwell was clearly frustrated, and he is taking a stance, even though he admits that he may lose a few friends and supporters along the way. Hartwell, with ASU's president, Michael M. Crow, recently published a scorching critique of the NIH on Bloomberg.com. The article was written with Dennis Cortese, emeritus president and chief executive officer of the Mayo Clinic.

Crow, the former executive vice provost at Columbia University and the founding director of Columbia's Earth Institute, had arrived on the ASU campus as president in 2002. He brought a seriousness of purpose and intellectual energy previously unimaginable in this sunbaked desert metropolis where temperatures hover above one hundred degrees for half of the school year and throughout the summer months. Physically, he seemed rumpled and awkward—he looked more like a college's football coach than its president— but he was riveting when he began to speak. Extemporaneously articulate and brimming with ideas about everything—science, technology, the economy, the arts, culture—Crow expressed his ideas with a booming voice and waving arms and captivated his listeners as he described his vision of "the New American University." In a 2008 article, *Newsweek* magazine said that Crow was overseeing "one of the most radical redesigns in higher learning since the modern research university took shape in nineteenth century Germany."

Hartwell, Crow and Cortese's article comprised a response to a proposal by Francis Collins to add a twenty-eighth subdivision to the NIH—a National Center for Advancing Translational Sciences—an idea which, in some ways, would seem to benefit the personalized medicine movement by helping to transfer findings from laboratories to the clinical setting. But Crow, Cortese and Hartwell argued for simplifying rather than complicating the NIH, urging Collins and the NIH to go back to basics, so to speak. The NIH, they said, was already far too sprawling, and they suggested, instead, a massive realignment to replace the present twenty-seven subdivisions with just three: A biomedical systems research institute that would maximize the impact of lab-based findings by integrating research from behavioral, sociological and environmental perspectives; an institute for health outcomes that would combine research and clinical insights to help determine which treatments work best; and an institute for health transformation that would develop new strategies to make healthcare more efficient and less expensive in the long run. If, in this third institute, they were also talking about developing a system of communication to connect the patient with the doctor and the scientist, it could be a very important addition. Steve Murphy, Saks, Camacho and many other physicians and patients would certainly confirm the need for such a system, and would take advantage of the opportunity to participate, learn and make an impact.

Hartwell, Crow and Cortese summarized their suggestions with a metaphor: "A simple way to characterize the fundamental difference between the present system and the one we have in mind is the push-pull metaphor. In the NIH's current model, fundamental science tries to push its discoveries on the healthcare system. What would work better would be a pull model, in which the healthcare system would identify what it needs and then choose the appropriate discoveries from basic science."

Crow, especially, has been biting in his criticism of the NIH, and his Bloomberg.com piece was not greeted with much enthusiasm by Collins or the research community. This resistance to change may not be surprising, for Collins is now probably the most influential and powerful scientist in the world. Why upset the apple cart? But Collins has always, at the same time, advocated change: of the system, of the way in which his colleagues think and of the way in which science and spiritual beliefs are merged.

What I find interesting about Francis Collins is that he is intellectually flexible and, some might say, elusive; he can maintain his beliefs, insisting that he has always been right, and yet deftly change directions. He is a former atheist who continues to believe in and defend the purity and clarity of science while insisting that God can make miracles. Similarly, he continues to explain the value and importance of personalized medicine and the impact of the HGP for which he will be most remembered by history, while at the same time refusing to buy into it.

In the summer of 2008, television talk-show host Charlie Rose asked Collins if he had undergone individualized DNA analysis—which was, at the time, all the rage.

Collins replied that he hadn't had such testing and didn't expect to participate in the near future. "I'm still waiting," he said. Surprised, Rose pointed out that Craig Venter had had his done—a full genome sequence, one of the first in the world. Considering the rivalry and bitterness between Venter and Collins, Rose might have realized this was not necessarily the most persuasive argument he could make.

"I am waiting to be convinced that we've arrived at the point where I would know what to do with the information," Collins replied.

Rose pushed the conversation further, pointing out that as a scientist, Collins should want to know the truth. "Knowledge is power," he persisted.

"Knowledge heals," Collins agreed.

"And yet, you don't want the knowledge?" asked Rose.

"I want knowledge that is attached to an action."

The interview continued in that vein, with Rose probing and pointing out the obvious benefits—for example, that the information might inspire Collins to change his behavior and lifestyle, if nothing else—and Collins insisting that the data available from those tests would not make much of a difference unless he could see proof. "I'd sure like to see evidence. I mean, isn't that what medicine is supposed to be all about? Not just saying, 'Okay, here is a possible way that you might use this information.' I want to know, 'Does it work? Does it change the outcome?'"

And yet, less than a year later, Collins had done the test—and he suddenly changed his lifestyle. He hired a personal trainer and began working out three times a week. And he improved his diet, eliminating most junk foods. (Friends say he was addicted to honey buns and fatty muffins.) Within six months, he dropped twenty-five pounds—all because he learned that he had an increased risk of developing type 2 diabetes.

What happened? Was Collins privy to new scientific evidence about diabetes? Unlikely. As a physician and a scientist, Collins was obviously aware that losing weight and exercising—and cutting back on the honey buns—could have many beneficial effects on his health. Most people who are not scientists know this, as well. Collins is not a poster child for personalized medicine. He is, rather, a fifty-nine-year-old man taking stock and preparing himself for a new job, as director of the NIH, to which he had been appointed by President Obama earlier that year.

And yet, the information provided by the test clearly pushed Collins to take better care of himself—an outcome that is terrific, but has little to do with genomics or DNA or personalized medicine.

Meanwhile, Venter has continued to be the maverick, pursuing his own private visions outside of the traditional scientific and research umbrellas of the federal government and the academy, raising his own money and resources and blazing his own singular trail—which he promoted all around the world, most prominently on nationwide TV.

In a dramatic scene on CBS's *60 Minutes* that aired in November of 2010, Venter removed a Petri dish from an incubator in his lab and held it up to the light. The viewers could see, inside the disk, tiny dark swirling specks of bacteria.

"This is the first synthetic species," Venter told interviewer Steve Kroft.

"It was designed on a computer, manufactured in the laboratory and gets its genetic instructions from a synthetic chromosome made by man, not nature,"

Kroft explained in a voice over. Then he added, "It's about as useful as the mold that grows in a bachelor's refrigerator, but scientifically it is a milestone."

"It's alive and self-replicating. That means it can indefinitely grow and make copies of itself," Venter explained.

Kroft asked if it was supposed to do anything or be anything in particular.

"No. We designed this just to see if we could do this whole experiment using synthetic DNA," Venter explained. "And now that we know we can do it, it's worth the effort to now make the things that could be valuable."

Venter, said Kroft, "believes this is the first baby step in a biological revolution, one in which it will be possible to custom design and reprogram bacteria and other organisms to churn out new medicines, foods and clean sources of energy."

Obviously, such an undertaking, like the HGP, will obviously take a lot more time, effort and resources than anyone, including Venter, could ever imagine. And it may well be that Venter will lose interest and turn to another scientific conquest before the biological revolution he is seeking will ever be achieved. He has certainly reversed his direction in relation to the entire HGP project.

In July 2010, a little more than a decade after the dramatic White House announcement, the German news magazine *Der Spiegel* interviewed Venter, and asked about the medical benefits of the HGP. Venter replied: "Close to zero, to put it precisely."

Did he think that there would come a time when the information we have garnered through the HGP would yield medical results?

"For that to happen we need a lot more information," he said. "Information about your body's chemistry, your physiology, your complete medical history, your brain and your entire life. We would need to do that a million times on different people and correlate that data with their genetic information."

Venter's feeling about the usefulness of the HGP has been echoed by a number of other scientists. "I didn't get anything useful from it, no I didn't," James Watson told a group of geneticists in October 2011 at the twelfth International Congress of Human Genetics in Montreal. The audience laughed when Watson uttered those words, but Watson went on to explain that he did have great hope for the potential promised by the HGP. "I'd like to see increasing numbers of children who have mental illness to be sequenced with their parents," he said, by way of example. Watson has a son diagnosed with schizophrenia. "It won't make their child healthy, but they won't have a double whammy of feeling like they did something wrong," he said. Any time such a child is diagnosed, "it would be immoral not to sequence them and their parents," Watson said.

Watson was speaking on a panel along with Seong-Jin Kim, a researcher at CHA University of Medicine and Science and the first Korean to have his genome sequenced, and a geneticist, Marjolein Kriek of Leiden University in the Netherlands, the first woman to have her genome deciphered. Kim's sequence indicated that he had an increased risk of macular degeneration, a disease that causes a gradual loss of vision. He said he was taking steps to deal with the problem through diet and exercise. Like Collins, he was going back to basics.

Kriek had decided to make her genome sequence public. One of her reasons was to educate. "It's not as scary as everyone thinks; it's a new nudity that people have to get used to," she said.

The last few days I spent with Murphy, watching him work, were filled with ordinary patients and rather mundane activities for part of the time. We visited three nursing homes for almost half a day; he had taken over a practice from a retiring physician and he examined and sat and talked with a number of elderly men and women, patiently listening to their difficulties and discussing their cases with nurses and social workers. Later that day, he gave a lecture about genetics to a local business club and then lunched with a vice president of research for a pharmaceutical company, discussing the future prospects for personalized medicine.

In his office in Greenwich, he saw a variety of patients, including a man with suspected prostate cancer and a man with severe arthritis. He also saw a physician who was now a medical administrator and no longer seeing patients. Whomever Murphy sees, he hasn't forsaken his dream and his roots. Steve Murphy always begins by taking a family history from a new patient—perhaps not as thoroughly as genetic counselors with their colorized, computerized charts, but thoroughly enough, he says. Murphy uses stick figures to draw lines between parents, siblings, cousins and grandparents and conditions and diseases. He scans the finished product into his computer. He won't treat patients until he learns everything he can about their genetic background—and he is committed to devoting adequate time to each patient he sees. Murphy has decided not to see any more than fifteen patients a day. In sharp contrast to the average patient-physician interaction of twelve minutes, Murphy will talk with patients for as long as an hour—and he often does.

Murphy's office is located in the town's historic Putnam Hill district in a century-old building called the Dr. Hyde House. A conglomeration of architectural styles and materials, the Dr. Hyde House is constructed of large boulders of random sizes, weathered beams and tan stucco with a roof of faded red Spanish tile. Murphy shares the space with a pediatrician and a nutritionist. On the outside, the stone structure is neat, but shabby; it shows its age—a look that pretty much reflects the feeling inside Murphy's quarters, which are practical and rather Spartan.

On a table in the waiting room are two stands holding Apple iPads, which patients are asked to use to fill in appropriate data while registering. It is all very conservative and well-conceived—Murphy is a man on the move, a physician on a mission, but instead of jumping headlong into a new and unexplored world, he is now taking it slowly, thinking before leaping and gradually infusing genetics and bioinformatics into his practice. Even his colleagues are beginning to take notice—and often referring patients to him, not necessarily for the genetic orientation, but just because he is a young, courageous physician with new ideas and plenty of time to spend with the people he treats.

One change that he has made—or has been attempting to make—is to pull back or perhaps retire from his Gene Sherpa persona. His blog posts are rather infrequent these days. It is difficult to tell whether he wants to continue or back out. These back- to-back partial postings recently appeared:

> In case you haven't noticed. I dropped off the blog radar for a while . . .
> But I am again back at it—

and

> In case you haven't all figured it out. Blogs are dead. Mine is too, sorta. I
> have less and less time to blog as my practice explodes. But . . . I am on
> Twitter, you can follow me there @genesherpas

And yet, Murphy told me, "If I were going to write a tagline about how my practice became successful, it would say 'It all began with the blog.'"

"But your blog is so irreverent," I said. "Your blog is not nice."

"You got it," he replied, laughing, "It is harsh—harsh and sarcastic. I tell it like it is—and that is what people want."

If Murphy meant that the public wants to hear from an honest, direct, down-to-earth doctor, then I think this assessment makes sense. But some of his posts came awfully close to not making sense at all—or showed him in a not-so-flattering light. Whatever the case, he's weathered the storm, and in a small but important way, has become somewhat of a change maker.

When I first started to write this book, I made a number of assumptions, beginning with Steve Murphy. I thought that Murphy and his attempt to start a practice in personalized medicine would be an accurate barometer of the future of personalized medicine. That is, I figured that if his practice prospered, so too would personalized medicine. After all, he was a doctor and so he had legitimacy; he was young, smart, charismatic and an entrepreneur, not to mention tech savvy. If anybody could take the next step forward, I figured, it was Murphy. But if Murphy's practice stumbled and died, well, then, that might indicate that personalized medicine had a long way to go to make a significant impact.

The fact that Murphy's practice survived and is prospering, but is not so much a personalized medicine practice anymore, I think, pretty well sums up the line between hype and hope—and between potential and progress—in personalized medicine. It is a sign of things to come, of those aspects of personalized medicine that may (or may not) be ready for prime time in the near future. Murphy is an innovator, not a game changer or a revolutionary. And he was quick to understand that science itself could not make the paradigm shift needed to make personalized medicine a household phrase because there were—at the moment, and for the foreseeable future—too many obstacles.

Murphy discovered that patients, more than any other group, were probably most prepared to make the leap into personalized medicine. Mariano Camacho and Michael Saks and tens of thousands of intelligent men and women, spurred on and supported by organizations like PatientsLikeMe and the 7q11.23 Dup Group, will gradually nudge the medical profession away from the hit-and-miss way of practicing and into the modern era, forcing the transition to a more thorough understanding and appreciation of genetics and the discovery and use of molecular diagnostic tools, like biomarkers and targeted drugs.

History has repeatedly shown how such paradigm shifts occur: experts tend to work at their own pace and sometimes with their own rewards (published papers, grants for research funding) in mind until they feel pressure being applied by the constituency their work affects. For example, in the organ-transplant arena which I observed through the 1980s and 1990s, insurance companies became increasingly less reluctant to pay those expensive surgical bills after dying children's images were flashed on TV every hour. Desperate parents lobbied their legislators through letter-writing campaigns and personal office visits, and by supporting opposition candidates. The development of AIDS medications ground forward slowly until citizen-activist groups like ACT UP, started by playwright Larry Kramer (*The Normal Heart*) were formed, and movie stars and rock stars, like Liz Taylor and Elton John, came on board to help pressure government and industry to stop procrastinating and take more concerted action.

This has not happened yet in the personalized medicine arena, perhaps because we are not talking about one disease, or a lifesaving effort for a particular group of people. We are talking, rather, about a radical shift of energy, resources, focus and philosophy in the entire healthcare system. Lee Hartwell and other visionaries are campaigning for a notion of sustainable health, and attempting to make an impact by involving all the major stakeholders—which includes scientists, legislators, pharmaceutical companies and the NIH. And, at some point, to be successful, they will have to add motivated patient pioneers to their campaign. This process will be slow but predictable, requiring communication, education, frustration and probably a little bit of anger and resentment, all of which Steve Murphy has repeatedly displayed.

In no way am I saying that Murphy is the only doctor who pays extra-special attention to patients or that he is the quintessential GP. I am only saying that sometimes scientists and physicians get so caught up in their research or the bottom line of their business practice that they minimize the reasons that they are there in the first place—ostensibly, to help the patient. To a certain extent, I think this has happened with genetics: the idea—the dream—of an "immense new power to heal" became, in the minds of scientists and public officials, something greater than could possibly be achieved. The White House announcement in 2000 precipitated major conflicting responses: Completely exaggerated prediction and expectation on the one hand and, on the other hand, a backlash from naysayers and resistance from many directions—spiritual, legal, economic and scientific. President Clinton may have wanted positive news to help him leave office on a high note, but the pomp and ceremony of the HGP announcement was premature. It might have been better to have noted and minimized the accomplishment until we could see more clearly what it might mean, scientifically and economically.

This is a major problem in relation to scientific and technological advances in this country. As Lee Hartwell has observed, we tend to celebrate accomplishments that make good stories and generate tremendous optimism before we conduct an analysis of the possible consequences: what a discovery might mean to the nation or the world or to individuals. As a consequence, it seems, we neglect to consider what can be done to shape the future, so that we are ready when the technology is ready. For example, Hartwell's idea of a national biosignatures laboratory makes, I think, perfect sense, and is an intelligent and thoughtful project to pursue to advance the personalized medicine movement and improve the healthcare system in the long run—but considering the economic and legal challenges, it is most likely pie in the sky for the moment, perhaps a half century away from being achievable.

We should be looking toward such a goal, though, and marshaling our resources to get there. What also makes perfect sense is to start to grapple with the legal complications that will soon be upon us—perhaps beginning in the laboratory and deciding how and under what circumstances we can have access to the information being stored there. Otherwise, before we know it, the lawyers will take over the personalized medicine movement.

So this is where we are as we struggle through the second decade of the twenty-first century, groping for answers. Our healthcare system is near bankruptcy, mired in a swamp of transition and debate; inconclusive, unfinished scientific investigations; unaware practitioners; and skewed governmental research priorities. And yet, there are many true believers, each moving science, medicine and healthcare forward in his own unique and vital way. Murphy, Evans, Saks, Camacho, Von Hoff and Collins are all on board Hartwell's personalized medicine train as it leaves the station. The train, as Hartwell noted, is "a slow train with a very long way to go." But as it switches tracks and makes stops at way stations, it will pick up more passenger: doctors, patients, scientists, legislators, executives and businesspeople who recognize the potential and promise—and, perhaps, the inevitability—of this immense new power to heal.

ACKNOWLEDGMENTS

Many people were involved in the preparation of this book. The authors would like to thank them for their patience and their generosity of knowledge, time and spirit. Without their help, this book could not have been written.

For fact checking of the manuscript and preparation of the Glossary:

Becky Bosshart, Sara L. Chadwick, Sam Gutkind, Robyn Jodlowski, Stephen Knezovich, Ginny Levy, Maureen A. May, Danielle A. Sharaga, J. Gabriel Scala, Chad Vogler and Kathryn Wells.

For manuscript review, editing and additional fact checking:

Leslie Rubinkowski, and most especially Donna Hogarty and Hattie Fletcher, managing editor of Creative Nonfiction, without whom this book could never have been completed.

Finally, the authors are grateful to the following people, many of whom appear in this book as characters, for their gracious cooperation and support:

Michael J. Becich, Michael Berens, Jonathan S. Berg, Michael P. Birt, Lawrence C. Brody, Kenneth H Buetow, Mariano Camacho, Michael F. Christman, Francis Collins, Sarah Coombes, Dave deBronkart, Michael J. Demeure, David Duggan, James P. Evans, David B. Goldstein, Hank Greely, Jeffrey Gulcher, Brad Halvorsen, Leland H. Hartwell, Tina M. Harter, Jamie Heywood, Eric Holzle, Joyce Ingold, Mira B. Irons, Gayle Jameson, Linnea Johnson, Lokesh Joshi, Muin J. Khoury, Bruce R. Korf, Joshua LaBaer, Eric S. Lander, Kim Lee, Kristy Lee, Gary E. Marchant, Deirdre Meldrum, Adam J. Messenger, Steve Murphy, Alan C. Nelson, Kenneth Offit, Jill Pitts, George Poste, William C. Powell, Jasper Rine, Jason Scott Robert, Cherie and Louie Ruffino, Susan L. Rutledge, Michael J. Saks, Daniel Z. Sands, Charles B. Seelig, R.F. Shangraw, Cécile Skrzynia, Amy Tenderich, Matt Tendler, Raoul Tibes, Jeffrey Trent, Daniel D. Von Hoff, Karen E. Weck, David Whitcombe, Paul Wicks, Raymond Woosley, Steve Yozwiak

GLOSSARY

Acidotic
Having an imbalance caused by an abnormal increase of acidity in the blood and other extracellular fluids. Acidosis is also marked by a corresponding depletion in alkaline reserves, and may be a symptom of uncontrolled diabetes, lung or kidney disease.

Actual risk
As opposed to perceived risk, the scientific probability of contracting a particular illness within a given time frame.

Allele
One of two or more forms of a gene that occupy the same place on a chromosome. Different alleles produce genetic variations on the same trait, such as eye color and height.

Alzheimer's disease
A progressive neurological disease of the brain that causes irreversible loss of neurons and intellectual abilities, including memory, planning and reasoning. Alzheimer's often is the result of complex interactions among genes and other risk factors, such as age and environment.

Amino acids
Organic compounds found in living cells that are the building blocks of protein. There are 20 amino acids; ten of these, called essential amino acids, cannot be synthesized in the cells and must be consumed as part of the diet.

Amyotrophic lateral sclerosis (ALS)
A disease resulting from the deterioration of nerve cells in the brain and spinal cord, and characterized by rapidly progressing weakness, muscular atrophy, spasticity, motor speech disorder and respiratory compromise. ALS is often called Lou Gehrig's Disease after the New York Yankees baseball player who was diagnosed with it in 1939. Five to 10% of ALS cases are attributed to heredity; the causes for the remaining 90 to 95% are unknown.

Apolipoprotein E (APOE) gene
A gene that provides instructions for making the protein apolipoprotein E (*APOE*), which aids in the packaging of cholesterol and other fats and carries them through the bloodstream. There are three slightly different versions, or alleles, of *APOE*: *APOE-ε2*, *APOE-ε3*, and *APOE-ε4*. The *ε4* version of the *APOE* gene increases an individual's risk for

developing late-onset Alzheimer's disease. People who inherit one copy of the *APOE-ε4* allele have an increased chance of developing the disease; those who inherit two copies are at even greater risk.

Autosomal dominant

An inheritance pattern characteristic of some genetic conditions in which the gene in question can be inherited from either parent, and only a single copy of the associated mutation is enough to express the disorder. Neurofibromatosis and Huntington's disease are examples of autosomal dominant genetic disorders.

Autosomal recessive

An inheritance pattern characteristic of some genetic conditions that requires two copies of a gene mutation, one from each parent, to express the disorder. Cystic fibrosis, sickle-cell anemia and phenylketonuria are autosomal recessive genetic disorders.

B-Raf

A protein that is responsible for helping to control the growth and division of cells. The *BRAF* gene, which produces B-Raf, can mutate, causing cancer. More than 30 mutations of *BRAF* have been associated with various cancers, from melanoma to lung and colorectal cancer.

Basal cell carcinoma (BCC)

The most common type of skin cancer. BCCs are characterized by an abnormal growth or lesion that arises in the skin's basal cells and can metastasize to other parts of the body if untreated. They are usually caused by cumulative or intense UV exposure, and can be treated by medication, surgery, chemotherapy or radiation.

Biobank

An organized collection of human biological material and associated information stored cryogenically for research purposes.

Bioinformatics

The application of computer science and information technology to the fields of biology and medicine. Bioinformatics develops and employs computationally intensive techniques, such as algorithms, pattern recognition, data mining, machine learning and visualization, to increase the understanding of biological processes. The assembly of the human genome is a great feat of bioinformatics.

Biomarker

Most commonly, an indicator of a change in protein levels that correlates with the risk or progression of disease. In addition, a biomarker can refer to a traceable substance that is introduced into the body as a means to examine organ function or health. It can also be a substance whose presence indicates a particular disease.

Biosignature

The term biosignature is sometimes used interchangeably with biomarker, but can also refer to the measure of several biomarkers together to get a larger picture of the function of a gene or a set of genes.

Bloom's syndrome

A rare autosomal recesessive chromosomal disorder characterized by extreme sun sensitivity, recurrent infections, short stature, infertility and increased risk for cancer.

BRCA mutation

Refers to mutations of either of the breast cancer susceptibility genes (*BRCA1* and *BRCA2*), which normally function as tumor suppressors. Harmful mutations of the *BRCA* genes produce hereditary breast and ovarian cancer syndrome, putting inheritors at higher risk for breast, ovarian, colon, pancreatic and prostate cancers. Because *BRCA* mutations are inherited in a dominant fashion, both males and females can express the mutation.

Canavan disease

An autosomal recessive degenerative disorder characterized by progressive damage to nerve cells in the brain, severe developmental delays, seizures and poor muscle tone.

Carrier

An individual who has inherited a recessive trait or mutation but does not express the trait or show symptoms of the disorder associated with the mutation. The term may also refer to those with an autosomal dominant mutation who have not yet developed symptoms of the condition.

Checkpoint genes

Genes that code proteins that regulate the cell division cycle. Mutations in these genes can lead to birth defects or cancers.

Chromosome

A structure in the nucleus of plant and animal cells that contains a threadlike strand of DNA and related proteins. Chromosomes carry the genes that convey hereditary characteristics. Human cells contain 23 pairs of chromosomes.

Context of vulnerability

The vulnerability of a tumor to a specific drug, as well as the patient's vulnerability to the drug. Ideally, a drug targets and decreases the cancerous cells in the tumor, with few side effects to the patient.

Copy number variation

Refers to an alteration of the DNA of a genome that results in the cell having extra or missing copies of one or more sections of the DNA. Copy number variations are a widespread and common phenomenon among humans, and are often normal variations without symptoms. Some, however, are associated with susceptibility or resistance to disease.

Crohn's disease

An inflammatory bowel disease caused by inflammation in the lining of the digestive tract. Crohn's is characterized by vomiting, diarrhea and abdominal pain. It may be caused by a genetic mutation, as well as environmental, immunological and bacterial factors.

Cyclopamine

A naturally occurring chemical, isolated in corn lilies, that causes birth defects, usually fatal, of the brain and eyes. It is currently under investigation as a treatment agent for certain types of cancer, including pancreatic cancer and basal cell carcinoma.

Cystic fibrosis

An autosomal recessive disease in which a gene mutation alters the protein that moves salt in and out of cells, affecting the cells that produce mucus, sweat and digestive fluids. As a result, these bodily fluids are thickened, and can plug up passageways in the lungs and pancreas. Most children with cystic fibrosis are diagnosed by the age of two.

Deoxyribonucleic acid (DNA)

Contains the genetic instructions used in the development and functioning of all known forms of living organisms. Different sequences of DNA's four bases—cytosine, guanine, thymine and adenine—make up genes, which are responsible for encoding proteins. DNA is found in nearly every cell of living organisms.

Direct-to-consumer (DTC) genetic testing

Genetic testing that consumers can order without the approval or permission of a physician or insurance company. Marketed directly to patients, these tests can provide consumers with their genetic information but not with medical recommendations.

Emphysema

A disease marked by over-inflation of the alveoli (air sacs) in the lungs, causing breathlessness and an increased risk of infection. The disease, which is generally caused by smoking, is irreversible.

Epidemiology

A field of science that uses biology, biostatistics and social science to study disease and health characteristics in a population. The cornerstone method of public health research, epidemiology helps inform policy decisions and evidence-based medicine by identifying risk factors for disease and targets for preventative medicine.

Epigenetics

The study of heritable changes in gene expression caused by factors other than changes in the underlying DNA sequence. These changes are brought about through marks in the epigenome, the cellular material that sits just outside the genome and can modify the expression of genes.

Epstein-Barr virus

A member of the herpes family primarily known for causing infectious mononucleosis. The Epstein-Barr virus is named for the two British scientists who discovered it, and may also contribute to the development of Burkitt's lymphoma and Hodgkin's disease.

Fabry Disease

A rare X-linked recessive disease caused by accumulation of certain fatty deposits in the body's blood vessel walls. The resulting decreased blood flow and nourishment of tissues eventually can cause bone pain, kidney dysfunction, high blood pressure, skin papules and decreased sweating.

Framingham Risk Score

Based on the Framingham Heart Study, the risk score is a calculation of an individual's chance of having a heart attack in the next 10 years, using a formula that factors in total cholesterol, HDL cholesterol, smoking status and systolic blood pressure.

Gaucher's disease

An autosomal recessive disease that results from an inborn error in metabolism. The disease results in an enzyme deficiency, allowing the accumulation of lipids in cells and certain organs. Symptoms include abdominal swelling, bone pain, bone disease and neurological complications.

Gene

The molecular unit of heredity in a living organism. Written in a sequence of DNA that occupies a specific location on chromosomes, a gene determines a particular characteristic or pattern in an organism. Genes undergo mutation when their DNA sequence changes. Humans have approximately 30,000 genes; each individual has two copies of each gene, one inherited from each parent.

Genetic discrimination

Occurs when individuals or groups are treated differently by employers or insurance companies because they have a gene mutation that causes or increases the risk for an inherited disorder.

Genetic Information Nondiscrimination Act (GINA)

A 2008 U.S. Act of Congress designed to prevent genetic discrimination by employers and health insurance companies. GINA does not protect against genetic discrimination for life insurance.

Genome

The complete set of genetic information for an organism, encompassing all hereditary material.

Genome-wide association study (GWAS)

An approach to genomics that rapidly scans markers across

complete genomes of many people to find genetic variations associated with specific traits or diseases. The variations identified often represent small risk factors for the development of multifactorial conditions.

Genomics

The study of the genome, or the entire sum of an organism's genes. This discipline examines the mapping of genes and the sequencing of DNA.

Genotype

The genetic blueprint of an organism that determines the outward, physical expression of a particular characteristic or trait (phenotype).

Glycogen storage disease

Any of a number of metabolic disorders caused by a genetic enzyme defect that results in an abnormal amount of glycogen (the storage form of glucose) in the body.

Haplotype

A combination of two or more alleles (forms of a gene) that are closely linked and inherited together from one parent.

Health Insurance Portability and Accountability Act (HIPAA)

A 1996 U.S. Act of Congress designed to protect health insurance coverage for workers and their families when they change or lose their jobs. Title II of HIPAA, known as the Administrative Simplification

provisions, requires the establishment of national standards for electronic health care transactions and addresses the security and privacy of health data.

HER2

A protein receptor located on the surface of cells that controls cell growth and cell division. Twenty-five to 30 percent of breast cancer tumors test positive for this protein, which leads to more rapid tumor growth and a worse prognosis.

Herceptin

The trade name for trastuzumab, a drug used to treat breast cancers that have tested positive for the HER2 receptor. The drug effectively blocks the receptors, thus preventing tumor growth.

Hereditary breast and ovarian cancer syndrome

An autosomal dominant inherited condition caused by mutations in either the *BRCA1* or *BRCA2* gene and characterized by a high risk of breast and ovarian cancer in women, an increased risk of breast cancer and prostate cancer in men, and an increased risk of melanoma and pancreatic cancer in both men and women.

Heritability

The proportion of observed variation in a particular trait (such as height) that can be attributed to inherited genetic factors in contrast to environmental ones.

Human genome

All of the DNA that a person possesses, which is contained in genes and stored in 23 pairs of chromosomes.

Human Genome Project

An international research project that began in 1990 with the primary goal of sequencing the chemical base pairs that make up DNA, and of mapping and identifying the human genome. A working draft of the genome was announced in 2000; the completed genome was finished in 2003.

Huntington's disease

An autosomal dominant inherited neurodegenerative disorder characterized by personality changes, loss of controlled coordination and dementia.

Hypoglycemia

A condition that occurs when blood sugar (or blood glucose) concentrations fall below a level necessary to properly support the body's need for energy and stability throughout its cells, leading to shaking, irritability, fainting and seizures.

Immunoglobulin

Any of a class of proteins in the immune system that combat infections. Immunoglobulins are commonly known as antibodies.

Inheritance pattern

The manner in which a gene is passed down through families. For example,

the pattern of inheritance may be as an autosomal dominant trait that is transmitted from father or mother to son or daughter.

Interleukin-2

A naturally occuring protein that stimulates white blood cells in the immune system. Interleukin-2 has been approved for the treatment of some cancers, such as melanoma and kidney cancer.

Ischemic heart failure

Either acute or chronic heart failure characterized by reduced blood supply to the heart, and generally caused by the narrowing of coronary arteries.

Joubert syndrome

An autosomal recessive inherited disorder caused by mutations in at least 10 genes and characterized by abnormal development of the brain, poor muscle tone, developmental delays, breathing problems and vision problems.

KRAS oncogene

A type of oncogene implicated in colorectal, pancreatic and lung cancer.

Leukemia, chronic lymphocytic (CLL)

A type of cancer of the blood and bone marrow, affecting white blood cells known as lymphocytes. CLL progresses more slowly than other types of leukemia, and is the most common form of leukemia in adults.

Leukemia, chronic myeloid (CML)

A type of cancer in which too many white blood cells, of the subtype myeloid, are produced in the bone marrow. Also known as chronic myelogenous leukemia, this disease typically affects adults; like chronic lymphocytic leukemia, it progresses slowly.

Lumpectomy

The surgical removal of a small tumor, which may be benign or malignant, from the breast. Also referred to as breast-conserving surgery.

Lupus (systemic lupus erythematosus)

A condition caused by the immune system attacking the body's own cells, and characterized by acute and chronic inflammation of various tissues. Symptoms of lupus include fever, joint pain, fatigue, skin rash and anemia. The condition is thought to be caused by a combination of genetic risk factors and environmental exposures such as sun exposure, emotional stress and infections.

Maple syrup urine disease

An autosomal recessive inherited metabolic disorder caused by the accumulation of branched-chain amino acids, which leads to the toxic by-product of sweet smelling urine. If left untreated, the build-up of these amino acids can cause seizures, hypoglycemia and severe brain damage.

Melanoma

The least common, though most deadly, type of skin cancer. Melanoma is typically treated by surgery, chemotherapy or radiation.

Mendelian genetics

A scientific description, originally derived from the work of Gregor Mendel, of how hereditary characteristics are passed down from parents to their offspring. The laws of Mendelian genetics typically relate to traits or characteristics that are caused by one gene.

Microarray

A genetic test that measures the expression of a large number of genes. It is used to identify duplications or deletions—extra or missing parts of a person's DNA.

Muscular neuron disease

Also known as motor neuron disease or MND, this term covers a range of neurological disorders that destroy the cells that control muscular activity. These disorders include muscular dystrophy and ALS, and can affect such essential functions as speaking, walking and swallowing. The cause is often multifactorial, and may include genetic, environmental and toxic components.

Mutation
A change of the DNA sequence within a gene or chromosome of an organism, resulting in the creation of a new characteristic or trait not found in the parental type.

Neurofibromatosis
An autosomal dominant inherited disorder caused by mutations in the *NF1* or *NF2* genes and characterized by neurofibromas,
or tumors of the nerve tissue.

Neuropathy
The disease or dysfunction of one or more of the body's peripheral nerves. This disorder may stem from damage to a single nerve or a group of nerves, and is most commonly caused by diabetes.

Noncoding DNA
Components of DNA that do not encode for protein sequences. Also known as "junk DNA," and originally believed to have no function, noncoding DNA helps control the expression of protein-coding DNA.

Nutraceuticals
A combination of the words nutrition and pharmaceuticals. The term refers to dietary supplements extracted from plants, purportedly with medicinal or health benefits.

Ogden syndrome
A very rare genetic disease, affecting only males, and named after the city in Utah in which it was identified. The syndrome, which is autosomal dominant, is lethal to infants.

Oncogene
A gene that can, under the right circumstances, convert a cell into a tumor cell. Oncogenes have generally been altered by mutation.

Oncology
The branch of medicine that deals with cancer, including diagnosis, treatment and palliative care.

Oncotype DX
A unique diagnostic test that examines the genomic profile of a breast cancer tumor to predict the likelihood that early-stage estrogen-receptor-positive, lymph node-negative breast cancer will recur in the next 10 years. This test also provides information about a woman's likelihood of benefiting from adding chemotherapy to hormone treatment.

Orphan disease
Any rare or ignored disease that the pharmaceutical industry has not "adopted" because it provides little financial incentive for the private sector to make or market new medications for treatment or prevention.

Parkinson's disease
A progressive disorder of the nervous

system that usually afflicts the elderly. The disease leads to tremors and difficulty with walking and coordination.

Peters plus syndrome
An autosomal recessive inherited condition characterized by birth defects of the eyes, short stature, developmental delays and cleft lip and palate.

Pharmacogenomics
The study of how genetic variation among individuals causes varied responses to certain medications.

Phenotype
An organism's observable characteristics or traits, such as eye color and height. Phenotype results from the expression of an organism's genes as well as the influence of environmental factors and the interactions between the two.

Phenylketonuria (PKU)
An autosomal recessive inherited metabolic disorder caused by mutations in the *PAH* gene and characterized by an accumulation of the amino acid phenylalanine. If left untreated, PKU can lead to progressive mental retardation, as well as seizures, pale skin and hair, and musty smelling sweat and urine.

Preconception carrier screening
Testing for an individual or couple that analyzes selected genes and screens multiple recessive variants

that cause genetic diseases, in order to predict the likelihood of offspring inheriting a genetic condition.

Pre-implantation genetic diagnosis (PGD)
An in vitro fertilization procedure for parents who have tested positive in preconception carrier screenings but wish to continue with fertilization. Only embryos determined to be unaffected by the mutation are transferred to the uterus.

Progressive muscular atrophy (PMA)
A rare form of motor neuron disease that affects only the lower motor neurons, or the nerve cells that connect to muscles. PMA often develops into ALS, which affects both the upper and lower motor neurons.

Protein
Any of a group of macromolecules composed of chains of amino acids, which are coded by DNA to be the building blocks of cells. Proteins are an essential component of muscles, skin and bones, and are required for structure, function and regulation of the body's cells, tissues and organs.

Proteomics
The study of proteins, specifically their structures and functions.

PSA screen
The acronym for prostate-specific antigen screen, a test that detects

prostate cancer by measuring the PSA protein produced by the gland. As high levels of the protein can indicate both cancerous and benign conditions, a biopsy of tissue is usually required for further diagnosis.

Relative risk
A measure of the risk to a group exposed to a factor compared to the risk to another group not exposed to the factor.

Reynolds Risk Score
An updated version of the Framingham Risk Score for predicting heart attack. The Reynolds score factors in two additional elements: family history and a measurement of the C-reactive protein, an antibody-containing globulin produced in the liver and normally found in the blood only during infection.

Ribonucleic acid (RNA)
One of the three major macromolecules (along with DNA and proteins) essential for all forms of life. RNA acts as a messenger, translating the information found in DNA into the amino acid code of proteins. RNA can also contain the genetic code for some viruses.

Sonic hedgehog pathway
A pathway, common to all mammals, that conveys proteins with a key role in the organization of the brain, ocular development and the growth of digits on limbs. Mutations can cause birth defects of the brain and eyes in utero, or cancer later in life.

Targeted therapy
A type of medication that treats cancer by interfering with specific characteristics of a tumor cell to stop carcinogenesis and growth. These drugs are called "targeted" because medications belonging to this class will not work on every type of cancer. Herceptin is a targeted therapy medication.

Tay-Sachs disease
An autosomal recessive inherited condition characterized by an accumulation of lipids in the nerve cells of the brain, leading to severe mental and physical disabilities, blindness and death.

Transcription factor
A protein that binds to specific DNA sequences, controlling the flow of genetic information from DNA to messenger RNA.

Translational research
Research that focuses on interpreting data obtained in a laboratory setting and applying it to a clinical setting. Translational research focuses on the 'bench-to-bedside' approach and can involve medical, behavioral or mental outcomes.

Triglyceride
The form of fat found in lipoproteins in the bloodstream. High triglyceride

levels can indicate diabetes or a risk of heart disease.

Tumor suppressor gene

A class of genes that codes for proteins that prevent cells from dividing too quickly or often. Mutations in these genes allow cells to grow uncontrolled, and can lead to cancer.

Type 1 diabetes

A multifactorial inherited chronic condition in which the pancreas produces little or no insulin, leading to unstable glucose levels and complications such as seizures, fainting and organ damage. This type of diabetes usually develops in childhood.

Type 2 diabetes

A multifactorial metabolic condition characterized by high blood sugar due to insulin resistance or insufficiency, which can lead to blindness, kidney problems, poor circulation, and slow wound-healing. Type 2 diabetes, which is more common in middle-aged and older adults than the young, is often caused by lifestyle choices, as well as such medical conditions as high blood pressure or high cholesterol.

Variant

A genetic difference among individuals, which may or may not affect the relative risk to the occurrence of disease.

Whole genome sequencing

The process of determining the complete DNA sequence of an organism's genome at a single time. A very small amount of DNA—such as that present on a swab of saliva or a single hair—is a sufficient sample for this process.

Williams-Beuren syndrome

A neurodevelopmental disorder caused by a missing piece of Chromosome 7 and characterized by distinct "elfin" facial features, developmental delays and cardiovascular problems.